How to
Lose Weight
Safely & Quickly

How to
Lose Weight
Safely & Quickly

Vijaya Kumar

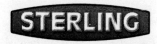

STERLING PAPERBACKS
An imprint of
Sterling Publishers (P) Ltd.
Regd. Office: A-59, Okhla Industrial Area, Phase-II,
New Delhi-110020. CIN: U22110PB1964PTC002569
Tel: 26387070, 26386209; Fax: 91-11-26383788
E-mail: mail@sterlingpublishers.com
www.sterlingpublishers.com

How to Lose Weight Safely & Quickly
© 2015, Sterling Publishers Private Limited
ISBN 978 81 207 5573 4
First Edition 2006
Reprint 2007, 2010, 2012, 2015

Printed in India
Printed and Published by Sterling Publishers Pvt. Ltd.,
New Delhi-110 020.

Contents

Preface

Are you fat or plump? Or just obese? Probably you tried various diets and exercises to lose weight, joined health clubs, aerobic classes, slimming centres, etc., but have never been able to get the weight off permanently. You find that the lost kilos have crept back almost as quickly as you shed them, comfortably settling down once again on the hips, arms and thighs. Don't despair. Reading this book and putting it into practice will work wonders for you, knocking off all that excessive weight quickly, safely and permanently.

It really does not matter what you did yesterday or ten years ago. It does not matter how old you are or how many kilos you want to lose. To achieve your target, it is important for you to set mini goals. Losing twenty kilos is extremely formidable, and yet making yourself five kilos lighter is not only attainable, but a goal you can live with for the present.

This book will help you to find the keys to success that exist within the framework of your own personality. The tools and information will help you to get there, but it is you who will do the work and reap the fabulous rewards to come.

Get started now and experience the joy of losing weight permanently!

Introduction

When it comes to losing weight and keeping it off, what really works? When we hear of someone who has lost weight and kept it off, we all want to know how they did it. What was the secret of their success?

Think of your weight loss programme as the most important gift you have ever given yourself. Enjoy the whole experience of eating, and get the most from every morsel you eat. Get beyond the idea that your life is all about your weight and food. While you are shedding off all that excess baggage on your body, gain the pleasures of those physical, spiritual and intellectual components that make you fully human.

The approach to losing weight has to be holistic: all facets of life are necessary and better together than they do alone. Diet alone is not the best method for improving your body measurements. The ideal method is a combination of a sensible diet to lose weight, and just about 10-15 minutes fitness plan of exercise to lose inches. The key to successful weight loss is making permanent changes in your eating habits, and your living style. Experience and study prove that weight gain is not a quick process. It is not a result of first days or months of overeating, but of years. So the safest and the most effective way of slimming is to lose weight sensibly — a kilo in a week is quick, safe and manageable.

Crash diets should generally be avoided as quite often they fail. This is simply because they just cannot be sustained. Moreover, people on crash diets develop a face that is gaunt and haggard, while their arms, thighs and hips are still bulky. The more severe the diet, the more you slow down your metabolic rate as the body is deprived of essential foods. This process can be dangerous if the diet is extreme or prolonged, or if dieting is repeated over several years.

While it is safe, permanent and ideal to lose about four to five kilos a month, it is very important to build health at the same time as reducing fat. It is also essential simultaneously to deal successfully with the causes related to obesity.

Various reasons are attributed to a person being overweight or obese, but a few that have been proved to be are as follows:

(a) Being overweight or obese can actually be due to some internal disease, and most commonly this is hormonal.

(b) Why does a fat person fail to use up as much energy as he takes in as food. It could be that though he eats minimally, some defect in the way his body deals with food deflects some of what he eats to his fat stores, and keeps, it there unused. This is because his metabolism is sluggish.

(c) In most cases, even with a low food intake, an obese person remains obese as his output is low. In other words, he needs to exercise a lot and expend extra calories, that is, he needs to correct the imbalance between his energy output and energy intake.

(d) In some cases, it is hereditary, but even in such cases, fat people can still hope to lose weight and be fit and trim.

Doctors often use a simple rule of thumb which gives them a general idea of the degree of obesity in people above the age of 25 years. With reference to a standard weight chart, you are clinically obese if you are ideal weight plus 20%. You are grossly obese if you are ideal weight plus 40%.

Don't despair when you stop losing weight after a certain period of losing weight. This is a weight plateau that most people hit, but this is just a temporary phase.

If you really want to lose weight permanently, you must feel strongly enough about it so that you will adhere to a sensible reducing-regimen, and adhere to it full time. You have to build up your will power.

Overweight is a major health problem to millions of people around the world. If you are obese and do not shed off that excess weight soon, your extra kilos can endanger your health and indirectly cut your span of life. You become prone to diabetes, high blood pressure, ailments of the heart and lungs, chronic nephritis, and so on.

Develop a reward system. Successful dieters have discovered that having something to look forward to at the end of each milestone helped to mentally and emotionally shorten the cycles of long-term success.

When you are setting your target weight, try to be realistic and not dream of a petite figure, if you have never been even once before you gained weight. The final success is the acceptance that there is bound to be failure along the way to reaching your goal. In spite of this temporary phase, gird yourself and carry on with your objective of reaching your goal. Remember, only you can get yourself off the couch to exercise, cook that healthy dish, and move that body!

According to a survey done by John Hopkins University, 67 per cent of the people diet to be healthier, 21 per cent to look better, 6 per cent for a better love life, 3 per cent for a better job, while 3 per cent do it just to be safe and healthy.

Chapter 1
Fallacies and Truths

1. **A glass of water in the morning helps to lose weight.**

   Many believe that by taking a glass of hot water on an empty stomach is a sure cure for excess weight, as they believe that hot water dissolves fat. Fat does not dissolve in water.

2. **Fasting for weight loss**

   Though some dieters fast once a week for weight reduction, most reported that fasting only caused light-headedness and deep feelings of deprivation.

3. **Honey for reducing**

   This is a fallacy. Honey has many therapeutic and curative powers, but unfortunately it cannot cure obesity.

4. **Bananas are fattening**

   Bananas are sweeter than an apple or an orange, yet they have only 85 calories. They are a wonderful source of potassium and valuable protein. They are filling and alleviate constipation.

5. **Standing while eating burns up more calories**

   This is a myth, for you tend to eat more while standing. Always sit and eat unless circumstances demand otherwise.

6. **Sleeping after meals makes you put on weight**

    It is not sleeping or resting after meals that makes you gain weight. It is what you have eaten for lunch or dinner that matters. Eat sensibly.

7. **Skipping breakfast is good during dieting.**

    Never skip your breakfast. Otherwise you will end up overeating at the next meal. After your dinner, your body has been on fast, and it needs fuel to get you going through the day. Eat sensibly.

8. **It is natural to gain a few kilos with ageing.**

    You will live longer if you stay on the thin side, and be successful in keeping at bay all the complications that set in with overweight.

9. **Too little calories help you to reduce weight.**

    This will be true only when you skip the empty calories that have no nutritional value. Otherwise there will be imbalance in your body, leading to a sluggish metabolic activity.

10. **Fruit juices are not fattening.**

    It is always better to eat the fruit itself than drink the juice as this gives fibre to your diet. It takes more fruits to make a glass of juice than can be eaten at one time. Readymade juices have glucose added to them, hence dieters should avoid them.

11. **Form does not matter when exercising.**

    Aerobics, weight training and cardiovascular workouts can have an adverse effect if you are doing them wrong, since you may end up using a different muscle than intended. You may also put unnecessary stress on joints.

12. **Potatoes are fattening.**

    Compared to bread or cereals, it is safer to have potatoes. Bread is twice as fattening as potatoes. Boiled potatoes are good for dieters, but not so fried potatoes.

13. **Saunas help in shedding off kilos.**

You may feel rejuvenated and great sitting in a sauna, but what you lose is the weight of water. Once the fluids have been replenished, the weight comes right back.

14. **Lemon juice is good for losing weight.**

While the vitamin C in the lemon juice helps repair worn out tissues, it does not destroy fat or have any action on it.

15. **Caffeinated beverages can energise.**

Coffee, tea and soda are stimulants that energise you quickly and then let you crash. It is therefore essential that you take an equal amount of ice water after the caffeinated drink.

16. **Margarine is better than butter.**

The man-made margarine has absolutely no nutritional benefits, whereas butter, a natural food, has anticancer and antiviral properties. Butter may even help in the prevention and treatment of Alzheimer's disease. The only benefit that margarine has over butter is that it is free of cholesterol. So use butter sparingly.

17. **Spot exercises can reduce fat deposits.**

Spot exercises only tighten muscles, and have no effect on fat.

18. **Vitamins provide energy.**

Many people swallow vitamin tablets in the morning, believing that they provide energy boost. The truth is that the energy is provided by the nutrients in the foods that are eaten. But since you are most likely cutting down on what you consume, some supplement is good.

Chapter 2
Tricks and Tools

1. Green leafy vegetables, juicy fruits and wholesome grains constitute a natural diet, one that is healthy and nutritious.

2. Sometimes you give in to temptation and eat what is forbidden for you. You will generally feel disturbed and guilty, and may want to abandon the diet for the day. This is not the right attitude. So what if you treated yourself to a goodie! You can still compensate for the damage by cutting the consumption of some other food item in your diet. It does take sometime to change old habits.

3. The key to successful weight loss is making permanent changes in your eating habits. Do not try to revamp your diet all at once. Start with a few adjustments and gradually build on them until balanced nutrition choices become a regular part of your life-style. Gradual changes in diet are more likely to become habits eventually.

4. Eat an abundance of fruits, like watermelon, papaya, apple, pear, orange, pineapple, etc.

5. Drink ice water. The body burns up 40 calories just by turning up its metabolism in order to warm the water.

6. Have an early dinner so that you have an hour or two to take a short walk after dinner.

7. Have a variety of food to choose from, and try to make it appetising, yet simple, wholesome and nourishing, keeping in mind the calories.

8. Drink plenty of water, and take low calorie beverages. These will keep off hunger, and sometimes what we often think as hunger is in fact thirst. Learn to recognise physical hunger.

9. Sit down when you eat. Be careful and watch what you eat while sitting before television, at the movies, while cooking or standing.

10. In between meals, when you feel like eating something, reach out for a glass of water. Don't gulp it, drink it slowly!

11. Take a walk around your garden, in the playground, around your block, etc., for 15 minutes. Sometimes it is just boredom or an emotional need you are feeling, which will make you want to give in to temptation and reach out for a food item that is taboo.

12. Use eggs as an inexpensive source of protein. They contain vitamin K, selenium and riboflavin. A large egg has only 75 calories and 1.6 gms of fat.

13. Celery makes a good snack choice as it takes up so much space in your stomach. It is a great fibre source and a natural cure for constipation. It also consists of calcium and magnesium.

14. Stave off hunger pangs with a bowl of soup. You can make a soup that is nutritious by using a lot of tomatoes, some vegetables for minerals, and a few beans for fibres.

15. Since you need to watch the nutrients that you consume, divide your plate into four quarters. Fill three-quarters of your plate with vegetables and fruit, and one quarter with beans, meat or dairy.

16. If you have a weakness for sweets, satisfy your sweet tooth. Choose a sweet like a candy or peppermint which has only 25 calories, lasts for quite some while in your mouth, and tastes heavenly. If it is a high calorie sweet, take just a bite. A taste is what you want, and not the calories.

17. If you must have a particular food, buy a small amount, and certainly not the big bargain size. Instead of buying a big brick of ice-cream, you can buy a small cup of it. If you are craving for fries, choose the smallest packet and take just a few from it. Give the rest away to someone nearby.

18. Choose red grapes over green, and Romaine lettuce over iceberg, as the deeper the colour, the more powerful are the cancer and disease-fighting antioxidants. The deeper colours are more tasteful, so eat more colourfully.

19. If you do treat occasionally to some sweet or fried food, do so at breakfast. Our metabolisms are more active during the day when we are more mobile. Our body is at optimal calorie burning in the morning.

20. Focus on deep breathing, into your stomach, and not just your chest. Oxygen is one of the keys to losing weight. After inhaling, try to take a longer time to exhale to eliminate the toxins from the body.

21. Chew your food thoroughly, and take your time over it. You will thus enjoy your food more, eat less of it, and the chewing will ease stress.

22. It may work for you better if you eat smaller meals, and more frequently, instead of three square meals. This depends on individuals, and you have to determine which suits you best, keeping in mind the factor of constant hunger pangs.

23. Learn to measure your food intake with your eye. Dieters are usually shocked to find out how small a serving really is when the diet demands just one chapati it means the size of your hand with fingers spread out, and not a 20 cm one! A serving of rice is the size of your fist, and not a heaped plate of it!

24. Many successful dieters claim that spirituality helps to finally lick the demon of excess weight. Turning to a higher power helps to turn off the voices in your head clamouring for food.

25. Sometimes, it is just better to get away from the house when your mind stubbornly refuses to leave the food scene. Just take a walk, or visit a neighbour, or do some essential shopping, but beware of buying those goodies that are satanic temptations to your diet upset.

26. You might try dimming the lights while eating. John Hopkins University reports that your appetite wanes under low lighting, while bright lights stimulate it.

27. You can always try switching your meals around. Instead of rice in the morning, you can have it at night, just ensure that the quantity does not vary.

28. Most people lose their invitation when they hit a plateau. Remember that it is only a passing phase, and so continue with your diet and exercises.

29. This may sound silly, but this secret seems to work when you are tempted to reach for that forbidden snack. Before you indulge your taste buds, take a deep breath, and count to 100. Usually, by the time you stop counting, your craving would have vanished.

30. That awful taste you have in your mouth when restricting calories intake can lead to eating. Instead, brush your teeth and tongue with a flavoured toothpaste to discourage snacking.

31. Another secret to burning away calories by at least ten per cent is by sitting upright rather than reclining. Good posture when standing also burns more calories than while slouching.

32. Talk to someone who is trying to make better — a colleague who is trying to stop smoking, a friend who has problems at work, etc. It helps to know that we are not alone.

33. Warm liquids like tea or coffee without sugar give your stomach a feeling of fullness.

34. While cooking, lower the heat so that you use less oil.

35. When a chocolate craving sets in, take a whiff of a strong perfume. This eases away the craving.

36. Try to keep your room a little chilly at night. You will burn more calories to provide the heat to warm your body.

37. Sleep deprivation can cause you to snack unnecessarily. So have good rest and sleep for weight lose.

38. You can allow yourself 200 calories a day for snacks that includes popcorn, jelly beans, 20 raisins, a cup of strawberries, etc.

39. Pinch your ear to lose your appetite! Surprised? Reflexologist believe that pinching your ear will curb cravings and lessen the appetite.

40. Flavour up your low calorie food with various herbs in both fresh and dried form. This will ensure that your diet does not become boring.

41. Believe it or not, researchers have found that just one good laugh is worth five minutes on the treadmill.

42. Remember that, when dieting, your body first loses fat from the areas you last put it on.

43. Without compunction throw away all the junk food from your kitchen. They do nothing to help.

44. Stay motivated. Never think of yourself as 'dieting', but focus on healthy eating.

45. Use small cups to serve yourself yoghurt, dals, curries or rice. Never refill your plate, or go for a second serving.

46. Cut down on the use of hot, spicy pickles. In fact, it would be wiser to banish it from your diet.

47. Take a glass of diluted buttermilk before meals. This will partly serve as a filler, and partly as liquid that is necessary during dieting.

48. Stock cucumbers and carrots at home. They are handy when you have hunger hands. They give you a feeling of satiety and they are low in calories.

49. Be always motivated. Think thin. Imagine yourself at the weight you would like to be, dressed in clothes that you have always wanted to wear. Now picture how others will react to you at your new weight. Enjoy the feelings these thoughts evoke, especially all the ways your life will change for the better with a slimmer, healthier body.

50. Start to care about your appearance while you are losing weight. Don't wait until you have lost weight. You will look more attractive and feel so much better about yourself.

51. If you are very fond of pasta or noodles and once in a while indulge yourself, have it only at lunch so that you can burn it off during the day.

52. Stay away from sodium. Keep your salt shaker out of reach for a few days to shed those kilos quickly. Garnish your food instead with lemon juice, pepper and herbs. Stay away from canned soups and soup packets, and also processed foods.

Chapter 3
Effective Diets

The basic principle underlying all efforts to reduce excess fat is reverse the imbalance in the body that is created when the energy expenditure is less than the energy generation. One of the most important remedial measures in this direction is dieting sensibly and effectively.

There are certain characteristics that make a weight reduction diet successful and practical. The diet should.

(a) Offer a wide variety of foods, including fresh fruits and vegetables, whole grain breads and cereals, low-fat or non-fat dairy products, and lean meat, chicken, fish or dried beans and peas.

(b) Be nutritionally balanced and provide a minimum of 1200 calories, unless directed and supervised by a physician.

(c) Include regular meals, at least three to six meals a day.

(d) Include snacks.

(e) Be based on personal food preferences that fall in the 'allowed' foods.

(f) Promote long-term habit change.

Sometimes, people don't look fat, yet are overweight. Excess weight can creep on insidiously with the passing years and can become a threat to your health. So one can be overweight without releasing it.

The key to both healthy eating and weight loss is to revamp your eating habits — eating more complex carbohydrates, fruit and vegetables, and cutting down on fat, sugar and salt. Sounds simple? But it works. The message that comes across loud and clear is that we should eat fat sparingly. Put simply—it is the fat in our diet that makes us fat.

Every time you take carbohydrates, your body uses up more than 25 per cent of these calories just to digest, absorb, transport and store the calories internally. But in the case of fat that you take, your body uses only 3 per cent of the calories to convert it internally. Our bodies burn carbohydrates and store fats.

Also, the same fats raise your cholesterol level, damaging your blood vessels, and possibly leading to cancers and other degenerative diseases.

Eating more complex carbohydrate foods and more fruit and vegetables is the quickest, easiest and best way to lose weight and eat healthily.

The healthy diet pyramid given below shows the main groups at a glance.

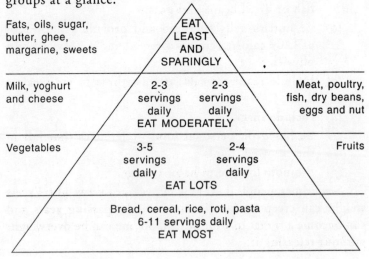

The idea is to eat most of the foods at the base of the pyramid, and least of the foods at the top, eating at least the minimum number of servings suggested on each level, and using the topmost level foods sparingly.

Provided meals are prepared from low calorie foods, satisfying and bulky helpings can be enjoyed. On the healthy food diet you will steadily lose weight until you have reached the plateau of your natural weight. And you will not gain the excess weight you were carrying before you changed your eating habits.

Eating the right food can actually boost your body's ability to burn fat. Severe rationing of calories in a diet makes it harder, rather than easier, to lose weight. Dieters who eat more of low fat foods lose weight more efficiently than those who eat low calorie menus with more fat. So the best advice would be to be aware of your calorie intake and cut down on fats.

Your complex carbohydrates will include rice, pasta, oatmeal, whole grain wheat, popcorn, corn and cereals. Fruits include apples, oranges, bananas, grapefruit and cherries, while carrots, beans, spinach and broccoli top the list of vegetables.

A balanced nutrient diet meets all the requirements of your body towards positive health. It is a sensible and practical way of eating for good health, losing excess body weight, and keeping the weight off when you lose it for ever. It is low in fat, salt, sugar, and cholesterol, and high in fibre, water and nutrients.

BREAKFAST

Never skip your breakfast. This should be the most sustaining meal, and should include complex carbohydrates to sustain your hunger. If you are trying to lose weight, and skip breakfast, you will probably be tempted into overeating later in the day. Many nutritionists agree that those who have breakfast work more efficiently than those who make do with a cup of tea or coffee to start the day.

Fruit, low in fat and a good source of fibre, can be very refreshing. You can try making a dry fruit salad for variation in diet.

You can try tomatoes, mushrooms or baked beans with wholemeal toast for an excellent low-fat breakfast.

Porridge is a good source of energy, and is very filling and satisfying.

A poached or boiled egg with brown bread is very nourishing. Or you can occasionally have scrambled egg or an omelette cooked in a non-stick pan, taken with some fresh bread.

A glass of fresh fruit juice in the morning provides immediate energy and vitality, and gives you a feeling of well-being, as they contain vital vitamins and minerals. You can have a combination of fruit and vegetable juice.

Proteins should be taken in moderate amounts, so take only a small quantity with your cereals like porridge or cornflakes.

You can substitute toasted bread for fresh bread, if you do not like eating untoasted bread in the morning.

Sample Breakfast Diets

1. *(a)* 1 glass of buttermilk (no salt or sugar), papaya or watermelon — a generous helping

   OR

   1 small bowl of cornflakes or porridge with a little milk and small slices of apple or pear for sweetness.

   (b) sandwiches filled with coriander or mint chutney and slices of tomato or cucumber

2. *(a)* 1 apple (unpeeled) or a generous helping of papaya or watermelon

   (b) 1 *besan chillah*

   (c) 1 toasted slice of brown bread

3. *(a)* 1 glass of fresh juice of carrot or orange or lemon (no sugar)

    (b)   an apple or a pear (unpeeled)

    (c)   1 yoghurt toast

4.   *(a)*   2 semolina *idlis* with 1 cup *sambhar*

    (b)   1 cup coffee (no sugar)

5.   *(a)*   1 glass orange or lemon juice

    (b)   2 carrot and cabbage toasts

    (c)   1 cup tea or coffee with minimum sugar

6.   *(a)*   1 cup tea (½ tsp sugar, if needed)

    (b)   1 toast (preferably brown bread)

    (c)   3 tbsps of porridge with very little milk.

    (d)   1 egg or 25 gms cottage cheese (*paneer*)

7.   *(a)*   1 cup tea or coffee (no sugar)

    (b)   an orange or lime or papaya or watermelon

    (c)   1 slice brown bread with tomato or cucumber slices to top it.

OR

I poached or boiled egg

8.   *(a)*   1 cup tea or coffee (with less sugar)

    (b)   1 egg with a slice of bread.

    (c)   2-3 tbsps cornflakes or porridge with a cup of skim milk.

9.   *(a)*   1 cup oats

    (b)   1 banana or apple

    (c)   1 cup skim milk

10. *(a)*   1 cup oats

    (b)   1 melon wedge

    (c)   1 egg yolk and 2 egg whites—omelette or scrambled with ½ tsp butter.

    (d)   2 whole-wheat biscuits

11. *(a)*   1 cup porridge made of ragi, a little milk and a small piece of jaggery.

     (b)   a small plate of soaked and sprouted whole Bengal gram (chana) or whole green gram (moong).

12. *(a)* 1 cup of tea or coffee (½ tsp sugar)

     (b) 25 gms paneer with 1 toast

OR

         1 toast with ½ cup cereal using.

         1 cup of skim milk.

13. *(a)* 1 cup tea or coffee with skim milk (no sugar)

     (b) 1 cup wheatflakes with ¼ cup skim milk.

     (c) 1 orange or banana

14. *(a)* 1 cup tea or coffee

     (b) ½ cup strawberries

     (c) ½ cup low-fat yoghurt

15. *(a)* 1 cup tea or coffee

     (b) ½ cup fruit salad

     (c) 1 toast topped with 25 gms cottage cheese.

16. *(a)* 4 egg whites —scrambled with ¼ cup mushrooms

     (b) 1 cup tea or coffee

     (c) 1 slice brown bread

17. *(a)* 1 cup tea or coffee

     (b) ½ cup cottage cheese

     (c) ½ cup pineapple cubes

     (d) 1 slice brown bread

RECIPES

Besan Chillah

    ½ cup gram flour (besan)
    ½ cup water
    ½ tsp chilli powder
    Salt to taste

Mix all together to form dough of pouring consistency. Spread a ladleful on a heated non-stick tawa. Turn when the underside is cooked. Cook the other side also, oilless.

Yoghurt Toast

1/3 cup thick yoghurt
2 slice bread-edges removed
1 tbsp each chopped onion and tomato
1 tbsp chopped coriander or capsicum
¼ tsp cumin seed (jeera) roasted and powdered.
Salt and pepper to taste

Tie yoghurt in a muslin cloth and hang it for 10 minutes. Add the onion, tomato and capsicum/coriander to the yoghurt. Mix in the cuminseed powder. Spread on the bread slice and sprinkle salt and pepper on it. Top it up with another slice of bread. Toast on a non-stick tawa without any oil or butter.

Semolina Idli

1 cup semolina (*suji*)
1 tbsp chopped coriander leaves
½ tsp soda bicarb
1 cup sour curds
½ cup warm water
¾ tsp salt

Dry fry semolina for 3-4 minutes on low flame till light brown. Cool. Add all the ingredients to it and mix well. Rinse the idli moulds and pour the idli mixture in them. Steam for 10-12 minutes. Remove from fire and cool for 5 minutes before removing the idlis.

Sambar

½ cup red gram (arhar dal)
3 cups water
1 tsp salt
½ tsp mustard

1 tsp sambar powder curry and coriander leaves
(1 lemon size ball of tamarind a Pinch of asafoetida (hing)
1 cup mixed vegetables (chopped). Pressure cook the dal. Cook
the vegetables. Heat 1 tsp oil in a pan. When hot, add mustard,
asafoetida and curry leaves. When the mustard splutters, add
the cooked vegetables, salt, tamarind extract and sambar powder.
Simmer on low flame for five minutes. Add the dal and cook
for another two minutes. Garnish with chopped coriander
leaves.

Carrot & Cabbage Toast

1/3 cup thick yoghurt
2 slice bread — edges removed
2 tbsps finely shredded cabbage
1 tbsp grated carrot
Salt and pepper to taste

Put yoghurt in a muslin cloth and suspend it for 10 minutes.
Mix all the other ingredients with the yoghurt. Spread this
on one slice of bread, and cover it with another slice. Toast
on a non-stick tawa, without oil, till golden brown.

SAMPLE LUNCH DIETS

1. *(a)*   1 spinach roti
    (b)   1 cup skim milk yoghurt
    (c)   ½ bowl of steamed sprouts with pepper, lemon juice,
            orange segment or apple cubes
                            OR
            ½ bowl sprouts with radish, carrot, tomato and cabbage
            chunks with pepper and lemon (avoid oil and salt).
2. *(a)*   1 cauliflower paratha
    (b)   1 cup yoghurt with grated cabbage and carrots in
            it (without salt).
    (c)   1 orange or banana
3. *(a)*   1 large bowl soup

    (b)   2 Marie biscuits

    (c)   Coffee or tea (if required)

4. *(a)*   ¼ cup grapes–pineapple cubes–strawberries in 1 cup yoghurt (sprinkled with pepper optional).

    (b)   Coffee or tea

    (c)   1 cup soup

5. *(a)*   1 slice brown bread with 25 gms cottage cheese.

    (b)   1 cup salad (tomatoes, mushroom, onions, broccoli)

    (c)   2 cups greens with pepper and lemon juice.

6. *(a)*   1 cup pasta

    (b)   1 tsp grated cheese

    (c)   1 cup tea or coffee

7. *(a)*   1 cup egg noodles mixed with 25 gms cheese or fish (cooked).

    (b)   1 cup spinach (boiled) with a little salt and pepper.

    (c)   1 cup tea or coffee

8. *(a)*   1 cup soup

    (b)   salad of 2 small cucumbers

    (c)   1 small bowl of cooked vegetables

    (d)   1 small roti

9. *(a)*   1 serving of fish or lean meat or skinned chicken

    (b)   1 serving of green vegetables

    (c)   2 medium-sized rotis

              OR

        1 cup cooked rice

    (d)   1 glass buttermilk

10. *(a)*   1 serving of sprouted green gram

    (b)   1 cup vegetables

    (c)   1 medium-sized potato (boiled)

    (d)   2 rotis

    (e)   1 cup soup

11. *(a)*   1 bowl raw vegetable salad
    (b)   1 bowl boiled vegetables
    (c)   1 roti
    (d)   1 glass buttermilk
12. *(a)*   1 cup pasta salad with vegetables
    (b)   1 cup cabbage (shredded)
    (c)   2 Marie Biscuits
13. *(a)*   papaya – generous helping
    (b)   ½ cup cottage cheese with chopped vegetables
    (c)   1 Marie Biscuit
14. *(a)*   1 large bowl soup
    (b)   1 slice brown bread toast
    (c)   25 gms cottage cheese
    (d)   1 apple or orange
15. *(a)*   1 bowl soup
    (b)   60 gms meat or 25 gms cottage cheese
    (c)   ½ cup boiled and dice potatoes with pepper and lemon juice
    (d)   tea or coffee
16. *(a)*   1 cup soup
    (b)   1 roti or ½ cup cooked rice
    (c)   1 cup vegetables
    (d)   ½ cup yoghurt
    (e)   1 orange or pear

SAMPLE DINNER DIETS

1. *(a)*   1 cup dal
   (b)   1 cup cooked vegetables
   (c)   a bowl of salad
   (d)   2 rotis
2. *(a)*   1 cup broiled chicken or fish

(b) 1 cup cooked spinach

(c) coffee or tea or iced water

3. (a) 1 cup pasta with 25 grms cheese

(b) 1 cup salad

(c) 1 cup spinach

(d) tea or coffee

4. (a) ½ cup rice

(b) 1 cup cooked vegetable

(c) ½ cup yoghurt

(d) 1 banana

5. (a) 2 cups spaghetti with ½ cup tomato slices

(b) 25 gms cottage cheese

(c) 1 cup buttermilk

6. (a) 2 cups macaroni with 25 gms cottage cheese

(b) 1 bowl green salad

(c) 1 cup soup

7. (a) 1 cup soup

(b) ½ cup salad

(c) ½ cup cooked vegetables

(d) 1 cup rice or khichdi

(e) ½ cup dal

8. (a) 1 serving meat or cottage cheese

(b) ½ cup cooked vegetables

(c) ½ cup salad

(d) 2 rotis or 1 cup cooked rice

9. (a) ½ cup sprouted green gram or
25 gms cottage cheese

(b) ½ cup green or leafy vegetables

(c) 2 rotis or 1 cup rice

(d) 1 cup soup

10. *(a)* 1 bowl salad
    (b) 1 bowl boiled vegetables
    (c) ½ cup cooked rice
    (d) 1 cup fruit juice or buttermilk
11. *(a)* 1 cup salad
    (b) 1 large baked potato
    (c) 1 cup beans (cooked)
    (d) 1 roti
12. *(a)* 1 cup salad
    (b) 1 cup soup
    (c) ½ cup pasta
13. *(a)* ½ cup dal or
        fish or meat
    (b) 1 cup vegetables (cooked)
    (c) 2 rotis or
        1 cup noodles
    (d) 1 cup salads
    (e) ½ cup yoghurt with carrot gratings.

The Right Fruits

1. When you feel hungry in between meals, reach out for fruits.
2. Papayas, pears, oranges, apples, watermelons, musk melons, pomegranates and sweet lime are good fruits. Bananas too are good but should be taken in moderation.
3. Mangoes, grapes and sapotas (chikoos) should be eaten sparingly.
4. Only when you have hunger pangs should you reach out for a fruit. Remember all fruits have calories. A medium-sized orange has 70 calories, equivalent to a thin chapati. Only fruits like watermelon and papaya

are low in calories, and high in fibre and water—
eat these generously.

5. Have 2 to 3 servings of fruits daily. Half cup of chopped or sliced fruit is equal to one serving.

6. Look for fruits that have a high water content, and avoid eating fruits that contain a lot of sugar.

7. Fruits like apples should be eaten without peeling them.

8. Papayas are a good source of betacarotene, a form of vitamin A, which acts as a powerful antioxidant, fights the free radicals that cause ageing in your skin, and maintains the health of your teeth, nails, hair and glands. So eat papayas generously.

9. Fruits are good sources of vitamins and minerals, and are outstanding for carbohydrates because of their content of natural sugar starches.

10. Place ripe sliced peaches in a bowl, cover with a tablespoon of yoghurt, and top with finely grated lemon peel—makes a great substitute for rich puddings, and tastes simply delicious!

11. Fresh fruit juices are good fillers in between meals. Or you can start the day with a glass of fresh fruit juice that will refresh you.

The Right Vegetables

1. Vegetables for salads should preferably be those with high fibre and high water content, like tomato, cucumber, bottlegourd (*lauki*), white pumpkin, carrot, raddish, and cabbage.

2. Tomatoes have higher calories than radish, cabbage or, cucumber.

3. Tomato has only one-third of the calories of onion, so eat raw onions sparingly with meals.

4. It is better to eat a large serving of raw vegetables and a small serving of cooked vegetables in which oil is used.

5. Ensure that you cook your vegetables in a non-stick pan, using a minimum amount of oil.

6. For added nutrition, steam your vegetables. Boiling destroys vitamins. Microwaving vegetables is also better than boiling them.

7. Use spices in your low-calorie diets. They are more desirable and satisfying, and they also activate your metabolism. So stock a collection of dried and fresh herbs and spices.

8. Sweet potatoes are full of vitamin A which is known to be a remarkable anti-wrinkling agent. The pleasing result is clearer, smoother skin.

9. If you do not have fruits at home to assuage your hunger pangs, you can eat tomatoes, Romaine lettuce, celery or carrots. You can steam green beans, broccoli or mushrooms and spice it up with herbs to make it palatable.

10. Capsicum produces heat to activate your metabolism and burns fat.

11. Parsley acts as a diuretic and is a nutritional aid.

12. A pod of garlic swallowed in the morning is beneficial in lowering high blood pressure.

13. Spice up your food with ginger which is reported to prevent and heal ulcers.

14. Do not add salt to salads. Instead, just add a squeeze of lemon or a dash of fresh pepper.

15. While preparing curries, avoid using pastes of cashewnuts, poppy seeds (*khuskhus*), sesame seeds (til) as all these have a lot of calories. Instead, for

thickening the curries, add a teaspoonful of soya flour, which also adds to your nutritive diet.

16. If you are eating out, for curries, do not take too much gravy. Try leaving the gravy behind as it has oil, and pick up the solid food.

17. Instead of taking a bowl full of cooked vegetables, eat an appetising plate of salad, or eat a few raw slices of carrots, which are healthier.

18. Keep a stock of mint or coriander chutney to make your low-fat meals tastier without adding to the calorie intake.

19. Add finely shredded cabbage, or steamed chopped spinach, or grated raw carrots to your raitas to increase the nutritive value of the curd without adding to the calories significantly.

20. You can enjoy a cauliflower or cabbage paratha without adding oil. Add a lot of shredded ginger, chopped coriander leaves and a green chilli to the vegetable. Add this to the dough and on low flame cook on a non-stick tawa.

21. When you prepare dal, add vegetables like bottlegourd or spinach to it to add to its nutritive value and fibre content.

22. Before seasoning your dal for the family, keep a cup of it for yourself. In your dal add some roasted and powdered cuminseed, coriander leaves and chilli powder. Red chillies are believed to increase your post-meal metabolic rate, thus helping in burning more calories.

23. If you are eating a curry that has both peas and cottage cheese, eat more of peas and just 2 pieces of cheese, as 2 pieces of paneer has 70 calories, the calories of 1 chapati.

Snacks

1. A cup of cucumber slices, which has only 18 calories, makes a very good in-between-meals snack.

2. Baby carrots or 1 cup popcorn can be a good filler snack.

3. A cup of fresh tomato juice has only 41 calories, and can stave off your hunger pangs.

4. A cup of strawberries is not only tasty, but is also low in calories (43 cals).

5. Celery is the snack choice of the world's most beautiful bodies, for it takes up so much space in your stomach. It is also a great source of fibre, and a natural cure for constipation as it contains calcium and magnesium.

6. Black grapes and herbal teas are great for snacking time.

7. Half a cup of yoghurt with 3 or 4 segments of orange is a nutritive snack.

8. An apple, a red one, helps to burn fats and carbohydrates more efficiently.

9. A cup of skim milk without sugar is a good filler.

10. A baked potato is low in fat and high in fibre.

11. Half a cup of sprouted green gram or any other legumes, with a chopped tomato is highly nutritive.

12. A glass of vanilla milkshake serves as a wonderful bracer between meals. Just add one teaspoon of skim milk powder to a glass of fluid skim milk, and add a few drops of vanilla essence. Add a few ice cubes to this and enjoy it! No sugar!

13. Instant coffee milk shake has the chromium requirement for an adult for the day. Mix one tablespoon of instant coffee with 1 glass of skim milk and refrigerate it. Shake it well before using it when hungry.

14. Likewise, you can have orange-lemon milkshake, using 1 glass of fresh skim milk, one tablespoon of skim milk powder, and half a teaspoon of grated lemon or orange peel, not forgetting to refrigerate it first.

15. Buttermilk without salt or sugar is a refreshing drink. If you like you can add crushed ginger bits or a dash of asafoetida to enhance its flavour.

HEALTHY SUGGESTIONS

1. A bowl of dal gives you 100 calories, but if you add spinach or bottlegourd to the dal to make it one bowl, then this gives you only 70 calories, as the vegetable has increased the volume of dal.

2. Brown bread is better than white bread. Calorie-wise, both are equal, but the high fibre content of brown bread wards off hunger pangs for a longer time.

3. Try having tea or coffee without sugar. In course of time you will develop the taste for it and will certainly help you in knocking off those stubborn kilos.

4. Take 2 Marie biscuits with tea in the evening if you feel hungry.

5. Avoid tinned foods. Take cottage and processed cheese sparingly.

6. Use a dash of dried mint, ajwain, shahi jeera or fenugreek (methi seeds) to spice up the flavour of your low-calorie meals.

7. It is better to eat 2 chapatis and half cup cooked vegetables rather than 1 chapati and 1 cup vegetables, as the cooked vegetables have oil in them.

8. When you feel like eating something in between meals, reach out for a glass of iced water. Drinking

generous amounts of ice-cold water is doubtless one of the best ways to reduce appetite and weight. Instead of gulping it, drink it slowly.

9. When you make alu-chana, take out some boiled ones for yourself. Boiled chanas are nutritious without oil, and the potatoes (boiled) are complex carbohydrates, and without oil, they make a good and healthy meal.

10. Listen to your body. Your body will signal you with what is wrong and what it needs. While some crave certain foods before the onset of their periods, some craving 'comfort' foods like pastries or ice creams or biscuits could simply indicate boredom or stress.

11. Never skip meals as it only sets you to overeat at the next meal. The key to sensible eating is to eat at regular intervals.

12. Always eat in a calm atmosphere. Loud and fast music, crowded places, thriller movies cause you to eat faster, and more. Always sit down when eating, and from on the entire experience of eating, thus enjoying every morsel that you eat.

13. Too much time on your hands often lead to mindless eating. So try to indulge in some other activity, like going out for a walk, or dancing to some tap music.

14. When you get tired, rest! A catnap is a no-calorie revitaliser!

15. When you make an omelette, load it with lots of vegetables as a delicious diet tool.

16. Pasta is a highly satisfying food that won't put weight on you as long as it is not loaded with sauce. It is easy to cook and store, and can be used in a variety of dishes, as it has a lot of starch, ideal as one of the slowest burning foods.

17. Instead of using cream use yoghurt.

18. Include wheat germ in your diet to get rid of pimples quickly and efficiently.

19. While choosing proteins wisely (lean meats, poultry, fish and egg whites), stay away from nuts and beans.

20. Limit your carbohydrates to two a day, and you will find the weight coming off quickly. Cereals and boiled or baked potatoes are the best choices.

21. Avoid carbonated beverages. Even low-calorie aerated drinks can give you a false bloated appearance.

22. Try to consume not more than a tablespoon of butter or oil in a day.

23. Include cardamom sometimes in your diet. It improves circulation and digestion.

24. Green tea aids fat metabolism and increases energy.

25. Fennel acts as diuretic that reduces hunger and enhances energy.

26. A generous helping of papaya aids digestion.

27. Vinegar is a natural storehouse of vitamins and minerals. Take two teaspoons of it mixed with a glass of water at each meal.

28. Add a lot of lemons to iced water to take away that awful empty feeling that cravings bring.

29. Eating between meals is not a problem. It is what you choose that hurts.

30. Drink less alcohol and always drink a glass of water as a chaser if you do drink.

31. If you are stressed out at bedtime, a glass of warm milk will help, for it contains relaxing amino acids.

32. If you have high cholesterol, take plenty of apples, carrots, capsicums, garlic, skim milk, oats, onions, seafood, spinach, soyabeans and yoghurt.

33. A glass of iced buttermilk (diluted) before meals is a good dietary item.

34. Use skimmed milk instead of full fat milk in your diet.

35. Instead of salad dressing or mayonnaise, use lemon juice, lime juice, herbs and pepper, and limit salt intake.

36. For dessert, take fresh fruit or low fat yoghurt.

37. Eat bulk foods rich in fibre and low in calories to help you feel full. Try to eat 50 gms of fibre daily.

38. Eats foods rich in calcium (milk, cheese, dairy foods, sardines) to keep muscles working smoothly.

39. Reducing fat will lower the free radicals that cause cancer.

40. Cauliflower, mustard greens, Brussels sprouts, cabbage, turnips and broccoli all contain a chemical called indole that helps prevent colon concer.

41. Apples, grapes, potatoes, oranges, lemons, oats, barley, lentils and chickpeas are goods sources of fibre, and they slow down the ageing of your entire cardiac system.

42. Drinking less coffee will keep your heart healthy and youthful.

43. Consume fish as a main meal at least twice weekly, but avoid fried fish.

44. Good sources of fish oils are tuna, salmon, sardines, mackerel, and herring whose nutrients function as anti-inflammatory agents and combat premature ageing and pain of arthritis.

45. Avoid special very low-calorie diets which have incomplete nutrients.

46. Limit your intake of a very high-protein diet which causes minerals to be flushed from the body, among them bone minerals.

47. Take plenty of fresh fruits and vegetables, for the boron in them guards your bones from weakening.

48. Bake, steam, broil or poach, but do not fry foods.

49. Do not stock junk food in your home.

50. Eat slowly, and chew your food thoroughly.

51. Swallow a garlic piece any time of the day, preferably in the morning. Not only does it help in warding off infections, heart diseases, high blood pressure, but it also makes the hair grow thicker and glossier, and also helps in curing chest complaints. It is also believed to stop the spread of cancerous growth.

Parties and Holidays

1. When you go to parties, leave the gravies, and pick up the solid food only, for the gravy has a lot of fat in it.

2. You don't need to skip the dessert. If there is any choice, choose the lightest one, and take a small helping. Enjoy every bite as you eat it very slowly.

3. When you are hosting a party, create a combination of choices of food so that everyone will enjoy your food. Have different combination of salads, low-calorie foods along with the other normal items.

4. Have a little of everything when you attend parties, so that you don't hurt feelings. It is not the food itself that is bad for you, but the excessive portions that are consumed.

5. Serve your entire meal on one plate, and no second servings.

6.   Eat your favourite foods first. The food that catches your eye first is the one that you should eat first. That is the secret of the perpetually thin person.

7.   Have a few glasses of water with lemon and a few carrot sticks before heading out.

8.   If you are offered 'starters', prefer steamed ones, else avoid the fried starters.

9.   If you have a choice of soups, take only the clear soups, for the thickened ones have cornflower that is fattening.

10. If you have to eat a Chinese food avoid eating preparations like Manchurian, for example.

11. Limit your intake of noodles or fried rice.

12. Avoid soft drinks, and stick to either fresh juices or water.

13. Prefer roti (dry) or steamed rice to buttered naans, parathas and kulchas.

14. After having enjoyed a rich dinner party, always remember to eat a very light lunch the next day—probably just a lot of fruits—to make up for the extra calories you consumed the previous day.

Chapter 4
All about Calories and Fibres

Calorie is the unit of energy. Calories are the main concern in any weight loss diet. They are contained in all foods.

There are four dietary components that contain calories: protein, carbohydrate, alcohol and fat. Protein supplies four calories per gramme, carbohydrates four calories per gramme, alcohol seven per gramme, and fat nine calories per gramme.

Weight is gained when you consume excess calories from any one or all of these dietary sources. However, a reduction in fat and fatty foods has the greatest effect on reducing calories in the diet. Choose a low-fat, high-fibre, high complex carbohydrate diet. In such a diet, fat constitutes 30 per cent of the total calories, carbohydrate 50-60 per cent, and proteins 10-15 per cent of the total calories. Weigh or measure the proteins until you can accurately estimate the size.

While a man of medium built generally spends about 2,700 calories per day, a woman of the same built spends about 2,200 calories. Depending upon each individual's nature of work, he or she may need more, or less, calories per day.

If you want to lose weight, it is generally recommended that your calorie intake should be reduced by half. If you wish to get rid of excess fat and weight, you should take 1000-1200 calories a day. Specialists never recommend to take less than the above amount. If you use up 2,000 calories in your daily work and take only 1,000 calories required by the body will be taken from the unwanted and extra fat of your body.

You have to be careful that your food is balanced and nutritious. While reducing fat and weight, you have to control the intake of calories, but also ensure that your health remains perfect. For this a balanced and nutritious diet is essential. You should have balanced amount of proteins, minerals and vitamins, reducing only the calories. It is also necessary that you take complex carbohydrates that is high in fibre.

The body fat of 500 grammes supplies about 3,600 calories, which are used as the source of energy. In a reducing diet, cutting down the calorie intake by half will ensure that a person steadily loses weight. Some mistake fewer calories for limiting the food intake. This is not the answer; you have to limit the calorie intake until it is less than the amount needed for the day to allow the body to use from the storage of fat tissues.

The chief value of fibre is in the fact that it is perfectly harmless and a laxative. Fibre seems to be natures best provision as a laxative. When it is softened by water, it becomes soft and pliable as a wet paper, acting as an emollient.

Fibre is generally divided into two categories. The less digestible bran fibre from grains and the more digestible cellulose fibre from fruits and vegetables. The fibre in fruits and vegetables are broken down to release nutrients. The fibre from bran supplied by whole grains passes undigested in the form of silky fibres through the intestines. Your body needs both types of fibres in your diet for good health.

The best sources of fibre are whole grain bread and cereals, raw fruits and berries, dried fruits, seeds and nuts, and vegetables.

Meat, dairy products, processed carbohydrates are zero-fibre foods, and in excess lead to building up of fat and cholesterol in blood, thus resulting in atherosclerosis (thickening and narrowing of arteries) and heart disease.

For a healthy diet, you need foods that are low in calorie, high in fibre, and balanced in protein, carbohydrates, minerals and vitamins, and also low in fat.

Popcorn is an ideal cereal food, full of fibre. Plain popcorn is non-fattening. It is also a complete protein, easily digested and thus superior to many breakfast foods. It is practically starch-free, and is a laxative, providing bulk. It is ideal as a snack.

CALORIE GUIDANCE

Food Item (100 gms) unless mentioned otherwise	Calories
VEGETABLES	
Brinjal	24
Beetroot, ½ cup	34
Cabbage (shredded), ½ cup	12
Carrot, 1 large	42
Cauliflower	39
Cucumber	14
Bittergourd	25
Raw plantain	66
Plantain flowers	28
Pumpkin	28
Cluster beans	56
Tomatoes	27
Tinda	27
Ridgegourd	18
Bottlegourd	13
Parval	18
Broad beans	59
French beans	30

Lady's finger	41
Peas	34
Turnip	34
Drumsticks	20
Coriander leaves (*dhania*)	45
Spinach	32
Mint (*pudina*)	57
Fenugreek leaves (*methi*)	67
Mustard leaves	55
Lettuce	23
Drumstick leaves	94
Colocasia (*arbi*)	101
Ginger	69
Onions	51
Potatoes	99
Radish	21
Sweet Potatoes	132
Garlic	142
Yam	79
Chaulai	46
Pumpkin (28 gms)	4

FRUITS

Apple	56
Bananas	153
Dates	283
Fig	75
Guava	66
Grapes	45
Gooseberry	59
Jackfruit	65
Lemon	57

Lime	59
Mangoes (raw)	39
Mangoes (ripe)	50
Melon (musk), ½ medium	37
Papaya	40
Peaches	38
Pears	47
Pomegranate	45
Plum, 1	30
Pineapple, 1 slice	44
Raspberry	55
Orange	49
Tomatoes (ripe)	20
Woodapple	97
Watermelon	28
Tamarind	283
Chikoo	118
Lichees	58
Passion fruit	36
Strawberries	27

DRY FRUITS AND NUTS

Walnut	687
Cashewnut	596
Coconut	444
Sesame (*til*)	564
Pistachio	626
Almond	655
Groundnut	549
Currants, ½	268
Raisins	319

CEREALS

Wheat chapati (30 gms)	70
Wheat paratha (60 gms) with 2 tsps fat	256
Rice, boiled, 1 cup	138
Barley	335
Riceflakes	350
Bajra chapati (30 gms)	108
Jowar chapati (30 gms)	106
Maize flour chapati (30 gms)	102
Corn	23
Cornflour	342
Oatmeal porridge, 1 cup	138
Wheat bread, 1 slice	75
Poori (16 gms)	68
Wheat biscuit	32
Khichri (140 gms)	238
Bread (brown)	218
Bread (white)	260
Cornflakes	360
Dosa (plain)	210
Idli	65
Idli (semolina)	8
Kachori	190
Noodles	390
Naan	336
Pasta	86
Puffed wheatflakes	320
Upma	260
Salted biscuit (28 gms)	127
Sweet biscuit (28 gms)	158

Toast	162
Ginger bread (28 gms)	108
Ginger biscuit (28 gms)	127
Macaroni (28 gms)	102
Sago (28 gms)	100
Soya flour	445
Spaghetti	375

PULSES

Black gram (*urad*)	348
Bengal gram (*chana*)	316
Bengal gram (*roasted*)	372
Red gram (*tuvar*)	334
Green gram (*moong*)	334
Lentil (*masur*)	346
Peas	315
Soyabeans	432
Kidney beans (*rajma*)	346
Raw sprouts	33
Boiled sprouts	18

MILK AND ITS PRODUCTS

Milk, cow's	65
Milk, buffalo's	117
Milk, goat's	84
Yoghurt	51
Buttermilk	15
Cottage cheese	348
Khoya	421
Cheese, 1 cube (25 gms)	50
Cream (canned) (30 gms)	71
Cream (fresh) (30 gms)	175

Skim milk, 1 glass	70
Milk (condensed), 1 tbsp	62
Icecream	96

FATS AND OILS

Ghee	900
Butter (1 tsp)	36
Groundnut oil, 1 tbsp	160
Til oil, 1 tbsp	126
Olive oil (28 gms)	264
Coconut oil, 1 tsp	270
Margarine (30 gms)	222
Palm oil (30 gms)	270
Sunflower oil (30 gms)	270
Dalda (28 gms)	262

BEVERAGES (NON-ALCOHOLIC)

Coffee, 1 cup, 2 tbsp milk, 2 tsp sugar	60
Tea, 1 cup, 2 tbsp milk, 2 tsp sugar	60
Cocoa, 1 cup, 1 tbsp milk	224
Apple juice, 1 glass	76
Coca-cola, 100 ml	40
Grape juice, 1 glass	92
Lemonade, 100 ml	45
Lime juice, 1 glass	47
Orange juice, 1 glass	72
Pineapple juice, 1 glass	82
Tomato juice, 1 glass	28
Milk with chocolate, ½ cup	167
Lemon juice (28 gms)	2
Lemon squash (28 gms)	36
Lemonade, ½ glass	6
Orange squash, ½ glass	39

DESSERTS AND SWEETS

Sponge cake (50 gms)	153
Chocolate cake	275
Orange cake (50 gms)	250
Custard, baked (150 gms)	200
Jelly (65 gms)	65
Pie (160 gms)	377
Boondi laddu (35 gms)	150
Carrot halwa (85 gms)	333
White pumpkin halwa (85 gms)	300
Apple pie (50 gms)	100
Banana custard (50 gms)	55
Gulab jamun (28 gms)	8
Chocolate (50 gms)	300
Fruit jelly (50 gms)	35
Fruit salad (50 gms)	35
Sweet pancake (50 gms)	160
Apricot jam (50 gms)	35
Pear jam (50 gms)	32
Pineapple jam (50 gms)	32
Fruit-yoghurt (50 gms)	55
Peach jam (50 gms)	55
Marmalade (50 gms)	140
Burfi (50 gms)	190
Pastry (50 gms)	310
Bread pudding	297
Chocolate mousse	139
Gujia, 2	387
Honey, 1 tsp	64
Jaggery, 1 tsp	56

Jalebi	494
Rice-carrot kheer	226
Sugar, 1 tsp	20
Maalpua	325
Lemon meringuepie	319

BEVERAGES (ALCOHOLIC)

Beer (100 ml)	25
Brandy (30 ml)	65
Gin (30 ml)	65
Rum (30 ml)	65
Sherry (30 ml)	43
Vodka (30 ml)	65
Whisky (30 ml)	65
Wine (red) (100 ml)	68
Wine (white) (100 ml)	76
Beef	234
Chicken	124
Duck	189
Fish	146
Ham	120
Lamb (breast)	492
Lamb (chops)	355
Lamb (cutlets)	370
Liver	145
Meat curry	162
Mutton biryani	276
Pork	398
Prawns	107
Salami	491
Sausage	310

Shrimp	86
Chicken roasted	200
Steamed catfish	120
Boiled chicken	210
Cod liver oil, 1 tsp	75
Lobster	120
Tinned meat	360
Minced meat (*keema*)	230
Mutton chop	280
Mutton rolls	120
Salmon	200
Crab	120
Fried fish	270
Trout (steamed)	110

EGGS AND EGG DISHES

Egg (duck's)	180
Eggs (hen's)	173
Boiled egg, 1	80
Cheese omelette	266
Egg fried rice	208
Fried egg, 1	107
Plain omelette	191
Poached egg, 1	74
Scrambled egg (with milk)	247

MISCELLANEOUS

Chaat	474
Ketchup	110
Batata vada, 1	118
Vegetable cutlet, 1	126
Sandesh, 1	57

Pakoras, 6	197
Rice *kheer*	141
Samosa, 1	472
Bhelpuri	182
Biscuits (home-made)	463
Dahi vada, 1	83
Dal, 1 cup	80
Chocolate Swiss rolls	337
Fried potatoes	120
Potato chips	240
Roast potatoes	120
Chidwa	350
Yorkshire pudding	240
Tomato chutney	155
Bread pudding	160

FAT-FIBRE GUIDANCE (100 PER GMS)

Food Items	Fat	Fibre
CEREALS		
Wheat bran	5.5	36.4
Cornflour	0.7	0.1
Custard powder	0.7	0.1
Oatmeal	9.2	7.1
Wheat flour	1.8	6.4
Wheat grain	2.2	9.0
Refined wheat flour (Maida)	1.2	3.1
Rice, raw	3.6	0.4
Rice, boiled	1.3	0.1
Pasta, macaroni	0.5	0.9
Noodles	0.5	0.6

Spaghetti	0.7	1.2
Bread, brown	2.0	3.5
Chapati	1.0	—
Paratha	12.8	—
Naan	12.5	1.9
Papad, fried	16.9	—
Buns	5.0	0.5
Cornflakes	0.7	0.9
Porridge, with milk	5.1	0.8
Puffed wheat	1.3	5.6
VEGETABLES		
Beans, baked	0.6	3.7
Beans, broad	0.6	6.5
Beans, butter	0.5	4.6
Brinjals	0.4	2.0
Chickpeas	2.1	4.3
French beans	0.1	4.1
Kidney beans (rajma)	0.5	6.7
Runner beans	0.5	1.9
Beetroot (boiled)	0.1	1.9
Beetroot (raw)	0.1	1.9
Broccoli	0.8	2.3
Brussels sprouts	1.3	3.1
Cabbage	0.4	2.4
Carrots (raw)	0.3	2.4
Carrots (boiled)	0.4	2.5
Baby carrots	0.5	2.4
Cauliflower, raw	0.9	1.8
Cauliflower, boiled	0.9	1.6
Celery	0.3	1.2
Cucumber	0.1	0.6

Garlic	0.6	4.1
Leeks	0.7	1.7
Lettuce	0.5	0.9
Bottlegourd	0.2	0.6
Mushrooms	0.3	1.1
Okra, boiled	0.9	3.6
Okra, fried	26.1	6.3
Onions, raw	1.1	4.6
Onions, boiled	1.2	4.7
Peas, raw	1.5	4.7
Peas, boiled	0.9	5.1
Peas, tinned	0.7	4.8
Capsicum, raw	0.3	1.6
Capsicum, boiled	0.5	1.8
Potatoes, boiled	0.3	1.1
Potatoes, baked	0.2	2.7
Potatoes, roasted	4.5	1.8
Potatoes, chips	6.7	2.2
French fries	15.5	2.1
Pumpkin	0.3	1.1
Radish (red)	0.2	0.9
Spinach	0.8	2.1
Spring onions	0.5	1.5
Tomato puree	0.2	2.8
Tomatoes, raw	0.3	1.0
Turnip, raw	0.3	2.4
Turnip, boiled	0.2	1.9
FRUITS		
Apples	0.1	1.8
Apricots	0.1	1.7
Avocado	19.5	3.4

Bananas	0.3	1.1
Cherries	0.1	0.9
Currants	0.4	1.9
Dates, raw	0.2	1.5
Dates, dried	0.4	3.4
Figs, dried	1.5	7.5
Gooseberries	0.3	2.4
Grapes	0.1	0.7
Guava	0.5	3.7
Lemons	0.3	—
Lichees	0.1	0.7
Mangoes, ripe	0.2	2.6
Melon, musk	0.1	0.6
Watermelon	0.3	0.1
Olives	11.0	2.9
Oranges	0.1	1.7
Passion fruit	0.4	3.3
Papaya	0.1	2.2
Peaches	0.1	1.5
Pears	0.1	2.2
Pineapple	0.2	1.2
Plums	0.1	1.6
Prunes, dried	0.4	5.7
Raisins	0.4	2.0
Raspberries	0.3	2.5
Strawberries	0.1	1.2
Sultanas	0.4	2.0
FISH		
Cod, fillets	0.7	0
Cod, grilled	1.3	0
Halibut, steamed	4.0	0

Sole, steamed	0.9	0
Anchovies	19.9	0
Herring, fried	15.1	—
Herring, grilled	13.0	0
Mackerel, fried	11.3	0
Mackerel, smoked	30.9	0
Salmon, steamed	13.0	0
Salmon, smoked	4.5	0
Sardines	11.6	0
Trout, steamed	4.5	0
Tuna	0.6	0
SEAFOOD		
Crab, boiled	5.2	0
Lobster, boiled	3.2	0
Prawns, boiled	1.8	0
Shrimps	0.8	0
Oysters	0.9	0
Squid	1.5	0
MEAT		
Chicken, boiled	7.3	0
Chicken, roast	5.4	0
Chicken, leg	3.4	0
Duck, roast	9.7	0
Turkey, roast	2.7	0
Venison, roast	6.4	0
Bacon, grilled	18.9	0
Bacon, fried	22.3	0
Ham	5.1	0
Beef, roast	28.8	0
Beef, fried	14.6	0

Beef, grilled	12.1	0
Lamb, chops	29.0	0
Lamb, cutlets	30.9	0
Lamb, leg, roast	8.1	0
Pork, chops	24.2	0
Pork, grilled	10.7	0
Pork, leg, roast	19.8	0
Veal, cutlet, fried	8.1	0.1
Veal, roast	11.5	0
Sausage, beef, fried	18.0	0.7
Salami	45.2	0.1
Sausage, pork, fried	24.5	0.7
EGGS		
Raw	10.8	0
White	traces	0
Yolk	30.5	0
Boiled	10.8	0
Fried	13.9	0
Poached	10.8	0
Scrambled	22.6	0
Omelette, plain	16.4	0
Cheese and egg	22.2	06
NUTS AND SEEDS		
Almonds	55.8	7.4
Cashewnuts, roasted, salted	50.9	3.2
Coconut	68.8	13.7
Groundnuts, plain	46.1	6.2
Roasted and salted	53.0	6.0
Pistachio	30.5	3.3
Sesame	58.0	7.9
Walnuts	68.5	3.5

MILK AND DAIRY FOODS

Milk, skimmed	0.1	0
Milk, whole	3.9	0
Milk, condensed	10.1	0
Fresh cream	19.1	0
Cheese, cheddar	34.4	0
Cheese spread	22.8	0
Cheese, cottage	3.9	0
Cheese, processed	27.0	0
Yoghurt, low fat	0.8	—
Yoghurt, whole milk	3.0	—
Chocolate Sundae	15.3	0.1
Cornetto	12.9	—
Ice cream, vanilla	9.8	traces
Ice cream, flavoured	8.0	traces

PUDDINGS AND DESSERTS

Cream caramel	4.5	traces
Milk pudding	4.3	0.1
Rice pudding	2.5	0.2
Chocolate mousse	5.4	—
Jam	0.1	—
Marmalade	0	0.6
Sugar	0	0
Chocolate, milk	30.3	traces
Chocolate, plain	29.2	—
Chocolate, white	30.9	0
Kit Kat	26.6	—
Peppermints	0.7	0
Toffees	17.2	0
Biscuits, cream	16.3	2.2

Biscuits, digestive	20.9	2.2
Biscuits, Marie	11.3	4.4
Cakes, fruits	12.9	—
Cakes, sponge	26.3	0.9
Swiss rolls	11.3	—
Pastry	40.6	1.8
Currant buns	7.5	—
Doughnuts	14.5	—
Eclairs	30.6	0.8
Jam tarts	14.9	1.6
Bread pudding	9.6	1.2
Fruit pie	7.9	1.7
Lemon meringue pie	14.4	0.7
Yorkshire pudding	9.9	0.9

FATS AND OILS

Butter	81.7	0
Margarine	81.6	0
Coconut oil	99.9	0
Corn oil	99.9	0
Olive oil	99.9	0
Sunflower oil	99.9	0

SAVOURIES

Mince pies	20.4	2.1
Dumplings	11.7	0.9
Pizza	11.8	1.5
Samosa, meat	56.1	1.2
Samosa, vegetable	41.8	1.8
Spaghetti	0.4	0.7
Tomato chutney	0.4	1.4
Ketchup	traces	0.9
Tomato sauce	5.5	1.4

DRINKS

Bournvita powder	1.5	—
Bournvita with milk	3.8	traces
Cocoa powder	21.7	12.1
Cocoa with milk	4.2	0.2
Coffee, instant	0	0
Drinking chocolate powder	6.0	—
Drinking chocolate with milk	4.1	traces
Horlicks powder	3.3	—
Horlicks with water	0.5	traces
Horlicks with milk	3.9	traces
Tea	traces	0
Coca-cola	0	0
Lemonade, bottled	0	0
Orange juice	0	0
Apple juice	0.1	traces
Grape juice	0.1	0
Lemon juice	traces	0.1
Orange juice	0.1	0.1
Pineapple juice	traces	0.6

ALCOHOL (per 100 ml)

Beer	traces	0
Lager, bottled	traces	0
Cider, dry	0	0
Wine, red	0	0
Wine, white	0	0
Wine, dry	0	0
Wine, sparkling	0	0
Wine, sweet	0	0
Sherry, dry	0	0
Sherry, sweet	0	0
Vermouth, dry	0	0
Vermouth, sweet	0	0

Low Calorie Recipes

1. Capsicum-Potato Special

150 gms capsicum
1 large potato
3-4 flakes garlic
3 tbsps tomato puree
1 tsp dry fenugreek leaves (*kasoori methi*)
½ dry ground spices (*garam masala*)
¾ tsp salt
½ tsp chilli powder
¼ tsp sugar

Method:-

Slit capsicums into thin, long fingers, Boil and cut potatoes into finger like pieces. In hot oil, add garlic and saute for a few seconds. Add the tomato puree and all the masalas. Mix well. Add the potatoes and saute for two minutes. Add the capsicums and mix well. Add ¼ cup water and stir for five minutes.

2. Vermicelli Idlis

200 gms vermicelli
½ cup semolina (*suji*)
1 cup thick curd
½ cup tomato sauce or ketchup
2 tsps chopped coriander leaves
3 green chillies, chopped
1 inch piece ginger, chopped
1 tsp salt
2 tsps oil

For Seasoning

½ tsp mustard

½ tsp cumin seeds
2 tsps chopped curry leaves

Method:-

Mix the salt with the curd. In 1 tsp oil fry the vermicelli till brown. Dry roast the semolina till the raw smell disappears. Grind the chillies, coriander leaves and ginger to a fine paste. Mix the curds, sauce and paste well. In the remaining oil, fry the seasoning and add to the curd mixture. Stir in the vermicelli and semolina, and mix well. Pour into greased moulds and steam for 5-6 minutes. Serve hot.

3. Peas Masala

1½ cup shelled peas
2 tsps oil
½ tsp cumin seeds
2 small onions, cut into rings, and separated
1 tomato, chopped
2 cloves, powdered
½ tsp turmeric
1" piece ginger, grated
2 green chillies, cut lengthways
1 tsp mango powder (*amchoor*)
1 tsp salt
½ tsp dry ground spices (*garam masala*).

Method:-

Boil the peas with a little salt. In hot oil, fry cuminseeds. Add the onion rings and fry till onions are transparent. Add the tomatoes and cook for a minute. Add all the masala ingredients and fry for 3-4 minutes. Add the peas and saute for two minutes. Cover and cook on low flame for a couple of minutes till done.

4. Tasty Toast

½ cup semolina
½ cup gram flour (*besan*)
2 potatoes, boiled and mashed
½ cup shelled peas
½ cup grated carrot
½ cup shredded cabbage
5 green chillies, chopped
3 flakes garlic
a small piece of ginger
2 onions
1 tsp salt

Method:-

Grind all the masalas and mix with the vegetables, semolina and flour. Grease a container and spread the mixture evenly on it. Steam for 10 minutes. Cut into desired shapes and toast them on a non-stick tawa.

5. Spinach Peas

½ kg spinach
1 onion, chopped
1 green chilli, chopped
1/3 cup boiled peas

For Seasoning

1 tsp oil
2 tbsps tomato puree
¼ tsp cardamom powder
1 clove, crushed
1 tsp garlic-ginger paste
½ tsp dry ground spices (*garam masala*)
½ tsp chilli powder
½ tsp salt

Method:-

Steam spinach with onion, green chilli in 1 cup water. Cool and blend in mixture. In 1 tsp hot oil, add the tomato puree, then clove and cardamom powder. Stir and add the garlic-ginger paste. Stir well. Add the garam masala, salt and chilli powder. Mix well. Add the peas and stir for a minute on low flame. Add the spinach and cook on medium flame for 8-10 minutes.

6. Nutri Khichdi

½ cup rice
½ cup green gram
2 tbsps red gram
1 tsp groundnuts, coarsely powdered
a pinch of pepper
a pinch of cumin powder
a pinch of dill seeds (*ajwain*)
½ tsp salt
2 tsps oil

Method:-

Heat oil and add all the ingredients. Fry for a minute, then add 1½ cups of water. Mix salt in it and pressure cook till done. Serve hot.

7. Bottlegourd Dal

150 gms bottlegourd
½ cup Bengal gram (*chana dal*)
1 onion, chopped
2 tsps roasted cumin seed
2 green chillies
1 piece ginger grated
2 tbsps chopped coriander leaves

1 tsp salt
½ tsp turmeric powder

Method:-

Pressure cook all the ingredients except cumin seeds and coriander leaves for 10 minutes on low flame. Add the cumin and coriander to the hot dal.

8. Cucumber Raita

1 cucumber grated
¼ cup curd made of skimmed milk
1 tsp chopped coriander leaves
a pinch of salt (optional)
1 green chilli, finely chopped.

Method:-

Squeeze out the juice from the cucumber. Keep it aside. Add all the ingredients to it, and mix well. Add a dash of lemon to the juice—makes a refreshing drink. You can also add a little beaten curd to the juice. The raita is filling, very low in calories, and very nutritive.

9. Brinjal-Soya Duet

400 gms brinjal
150 gms soya granules
1 small onion, chopped
1 tsp chopped garlic
1 tsp chopped ginger
3 tomatoes, chopped
1 tsp oil
1 tsp dry ground spices (*garam masala*)
2 tsps lime juice
100 ml curd, whipped
1 tsp salt
Capsicum or peas for garnishing

Method:-

Cut brinjals lengthwise into halves. Steam for five minutes. Scoop out pulp and chop finely. Soak soya granules in boiling water for a minute. Drain and keep aside. Heat oil. Saute the chopped ginger and garlic for a few seconds. Add the tomato, soya, lime juice, salt. Mix well. Stuff spoonfuls of the paste into the brinjal halves and steam for five minutes. Garnish with capsicum slices or peas.

10. Steamed Chicken Idlis with Date Mint Chutney

200 gms rice
100 gms black gram
Salt to taste

Chicken filling

200 gms boneless chicken cubes
100 ml low fat curd
½ tsp chopped garlic
¼ tsp chilli powder
½ tsp dry ground spices (*garam masala*)
½ tsp cumin powder
½ tsp coriander powder
Salt to taste

For the chutney

75 gms coriander leaves
50 gms mint leaves
2 tsps chopped dates
3 tbsp low-fat curd
2 tsps lime juice
1 tsp chopped garlic
Salt to taste

Method:-

Soak rice and black gram separately for six hours. Grind to a fine dough. Add salt and allow to ferment.

Mix all the ingredients for the chicken filling in a bowl and refrigerate for 15 minutes. Stir-fry in a non-stick tawa for 10-12 minutes.

Grind all the ingredients for the chutney into a fine paste, and chill.

Lightly grease the idli moulds. Pour 1 heaped tablespoon of batter in the mould. Sprinkle a portion of the chicken filling over it. Cover this with another tablespoon of the idli batter. Steam the idlis till done.

11. Cauliflower in Sauce

300 gms cauliflower florets with long stalks
8-10 flakes garlic, crushed
1 green chilli, chopped
2 tbsps soya sauce
2 tsps tomato ketchup
1 tsp vinegar
¼ tsp fresh pepper powder
2 tbsps chopped coriander

Method:-

Boil 3 cups of water with 1½ tsp salt. Add the cauliflower florets and boil for three minutes, but do not overcook, strain. In hot oil fry garlic and green chillies for a few seconds. On low heat, add the soya and tomato sauces, and vinegar. Cook for a few seconds. Add the coriander. Stir for half a minute. Add 2-3 tablespoons of water. Boil for a minute. Add the cauliflower and pepper. Stir-fry for five minutes. Serve hot.

12. Peppery Moong

1 cup whole green gram (*moong*)
2 tsps black pepper
½ cup grated coconut
2 tsps Bengal gram
2 tsps coriander seeds
½ tsp salt
1 tsp grated cheese

Method:-

Roast the Bengal gram and coriander. Grind them along with the pepper and coconut to a fine paste. Put the green gram in a container in the pressure cooker. Add 2 cups of water, coconut paste and salt. Cook for 10 minutes. Serve hot with grated cheese sprinkled over it.

13. Chana-Potato with Chutney

2 potatoes, boiled
½ cup boiled chick peas (*kabuli chana*)
2-3 tbsps chopped coriander leaves

Chutney

1 tbsp mango powder (*amchoor*)
1½ tbsps sugar
3/4 tsp salt
3/4 tsp cumin powder (*roasted*)
½ cup water
1½ tsps refined flour (*maida*) dissolved in a little water.

Method:-

Cube the potatoes into half-inch pieces. Mix together the amchoor, sugar, salt, chilli powder, cumin powder and water. Boil for a minute, add the water-dissolved maida, and stir continuously. Boil on low flame for three minutes. Remove from fire. Mix in the boiled potatoes, boiled chanas and coriander leaves.

14. Stuffed Tomatoes

    4 large and firm tomatoes

For the filling

    200 gms prawns, shelled and deveined
    2 tsps ginger-garlic-green chilli paste
    2 tsps chopped coriander leaves
    2 tsps grated cheese
    1 tsp oil

Method:-

Cut the stem end of each tomato. Invert them to drain, after scooping out the pulp. Chop the pulp finely. Mix all the filling ingredients and saute in oil for five minutes. Stuff the tomatoes with the filling, and seal the opening with the cut slice. Steam for five minutes Serve hot with rotis.

15. Apple-Cucumber Shake

    2 apples
    4 slices of cucumber
    1 tsp lemon juice
    ½ glass iced water

Method:-

Cut the apples into small chunks. Put them in a blender along with lemon juice and cucumber. Run the blender till there are no lumps in the juice. Blend with iced water. A refreshing drink low in calories.

16. Cucumber Chutney

    1 cucumber, sliced
    a small piece of ginger

a few coriander leaves
1 green chilli
salt to taste
1 tsp lemon juice

Method:-

Mix together all the ingredients in a blender. Run the blender for a minute. Serve with toast or brown bread slice.

17. Spicy Cauliflower

500 gms cauliflower, cut into florets
2 tsps oil
½ tsp cumin seeds
1 tbsp dry fenugreek leaves (*kasoori methi*)
1 piece ginger, cut into juliennes

For the marinade

3/4 cup thick curd
2 tsps ginger-garlic paste
1 tsp salt
3/4 tsp chilli powder
½ tsp roasted cumin powder
¼ tsp rock salt

Method:-

Boil 4 cups of water with 1 tsp salt. Add cauliflower to the boiling water and boil for three minutes. Mix all the ingredients together for the marinade. Coat all the florets with this, and leave aside for half an hour. In hot oil fry cumin. Add the cauliflower. Mix well. Add the kasoori methi and ginger julienne. Fry for five minutes. Serve hot.

18. Hot Vegetable Juice

1 bunch spinach
1 tomato (large)

1 flake garlic
1 piece ginger
pepper and salt to taste

Method:-

Put together the spinach, tomato, the garlic-ginger pieces, and the salt and pepper in a vessel. Add 1 cup water. Steam for three minutes. Run it in a blender, and serve hot.

19. Dieter's Delight

2 ripe bananas, mashed
1 cup grated pineapple
1 cup grated apple
1 cup orange juice
1 tin unsweetened condensed milk
1 tbsp honey
2 tsps crushed raisins

Method:-

Mix all the ingredients well. Grease a container and pour the contents into it. Cover it with an aluminium foil and tie it securely with a string. Steam it for 15 minutes. Cool and then chill it. Serve with fruit chunks on it.

20. Mushroom Curry

200 gms mushrooms, washed
4 tbsps tomato puree
½ cup chopped coriander
½ tsp dill seeds (*ajwain*)
1 piece ginger julienne
2 green chillies, chopped
½ tsp mango powder (*amchoor*)
1 tsp sugar
½ tsp dry ground spices (*garam masala*)
¼ tsp chilli powder

2 tsps coriander powder

1 tsp salt

Method:-

Cut the stem into round slices. In hot oil fry the ajwain. Add the green chillies and ginger, and stir for a minute. Add the puree. Then add the chilli powder, coriander powder, amchoor, sugar, garam masala and salt. Fry for a minute. Add water, then add the mushrooms and the stem. Cook for 10-15 minutes till the mushrooms are done. Add the coriander leaves, and 2-3 tablespoons of water. Boil for another two minutes. Serve hot.

21. Pineapple Cocktail

1 glass of fresh pineapple juice

1 apple, cubed

1 tsp honey

2 cherries

Method:-

Run all the ingredients, except cherries in a blender. Decorate it with cherries and serve chilled.

22. Spicy Beans

200 gms french beans, chopped

1 tomato, cut lengthwise

2 tbsps dry fenugreek leaves (*kasoori methi*)

1 tsp mustard

2 tsps oil

For the spice mixture

4 tbsps curd

4 tbsps coriander leaves, chopped

1 tsp cumin seeds

1 tsp coriander powder

3/4 tsp chilli powder
2 flakes garlic, chopped
½ piece ginger
¼ tsp turmeric powder
1 tsp salt

Method:-

Grind together the coriander leaves, coriander powder, cumin seeds, chilli powder, garlic, ginger, salt and turmeric with curd in a blender to a fine paste. In hot oil, splutter the mustard. Add the beans. Cover and cook on low flame for 10 minutes, stirring regularly. Add the spice mixture and kasoori methi. Fry on medium flame for five minutes, stirring occasionally. Add the tomato pieces, and stir-fry for a minute. Serve hot.

23. Spinach Dal

1½ cups chopped spinach
½ cup red gram
1 flake garlic, chopped
½ piece ginger, chopped
1 green chilli, chopped
½ tsp turmeric powder
1 tsp salt
1½ tsps roasted cumin powder.

Method:-

Mix all the ingredients except cumin in a vessel. Pressure cook. Remove the vessel from the cooker. Add the cumin powder, and serve hot with chapati or rice.

24. Apple crisp

4 apples, sliced
1/3 cup brown sugar
¼ cup wheat flour (*gehun ka atta*)

¼ cup oats

1 tsp cinnamon powder

2 tbsps butter, softened

Method:-

Preheat oven 375°F. Grease an 8×8 inch pan. Place apple slices in it. Mix together all the ingredients and sprinkle over apples. Bake for 30 minutes, or until apples are crisp.

25. Delicious Brinjals

250 gms round, small brinjals

4 tbsps tomato puree

½ tsp cumin seeds

6 flakes garlic, chopped

½ tsp dill seeds (*ajwain*)

For masala

1¼ tsp salt

3 tsps coriander powder

3/4 tsp dry ground spices (*garam masala*)

1½ tsps mango powder (*amchoor*)

3/4 tsp turmeric powder

Method:-

Make four slits in each brinjal, halfway, but not till the end. Mix the masala ingredients and fill in each brinjal in the slits. In hot oil, add the cumin and ajwain. When the cumin splutters, add the tomato puree and cook for a minute. Add the brinjals, and the masala, if any is left over. Mix well. Cook covered for about 20 minutes on very low flame till brinjals are soft.

Chapter 5
Exercises

Exercise is essential to the success of a weight loss and weight maintenance programme. Weight loss programmes that incorporate exercise with diet are more effective than diet alone. Permanent weight loss, or more precisely fat loss, can only occur with the combination of diet and exercise.

A well-planned fitness programme should include exercises for the entire body, working the muscles from head to toe, You can rest assured that you will lose inches from the right places by exercising the right parts of your body.

With some slimming foods offering miracle weight loss without exercise, and some fitness plans offering quick weight loss without dieting, it is easy to see why people think that you can diet without exercising or exercise without dieting. But the answer is not that simple. If you want to get fit, lose weight and maintain your fitness and weight loss for the rest of your life, then you need to diet and exercise. Most people fail on diets because the diets are temporary, unpleasant and nutritionally unsound. The diets leave you feeling deprived, bad tempered, depressed and yes—hungry.

But don't despair. Research now shows that adding exercise to a moderate diet is a far more effective way to lose weight than alone. Moderation is the key to successful dieting and exercise. Moderate exercise with a moderate plan is the easiest and quickest way to lose those unwanted pounds and keep them off forever.

The gradual weight loss that results from a change in eating and exercise habits is more likely to be a permanent loss and one that is most beneficial to health. All we need to do is to strike the right balance between all the factors affecting health and fitness, between activity and rest, between work and recreation, between essential nutrients and tasty treats.

What is needed is an enjoyable session of exercise two or three times a week for your heart, lungs and general circulatory system. The key word is *enjoyable*. If it is not enjoyable you are not likely to persevere with it, and the more enjoyable it is the more benefit you are likely to derive from it.

We don't have to punish the body with gruelling routines for everyday fitness, or sweat to a state of near exhaustion. Exercise must be a joy. There is a 'play-way' to fitness for everyday life. Avoid the possibility of monotony and subsequent boredom. Don't be housebound, it leads to sitting around.

Exercise is enjoyable, easily incorporated into your life-style, cost-free, and guaranteed to affect your health in a positive way. Weight loss at first will depend upon how overweight you are, the rigorous nature of the exercise taken, and diet control. Do not be surprised if you loss more than a kilo of weight in the first week. Not all of this will be fat, there will be loss of water also. After this there will be a gradual loss. You might hit the plateau when your weight refuses to budge. Don't despair, but continue with your exercises and diet, and soon you will once again see all those kilos being shed off.

There is no age for exercises. Your body can be rejuvenated at any time in your life. Whether you are middle-aged or pushing 70, you can regain the vigour, vitality and muscular strength that you thought were gone forever.

Devote about 15 minutes every day for exercises. The exercises should be started very slowly, with a gradual increase in speed and vigour. Do not strain yourself, if you get tired after doing an exercise four or five times. Go on to the next one, soon you will be able to do them with ease. Put on your favourite music and enjoy doing these simple exercises.

Warm-ups and Cool Downs

Warm-ups and cool-downs are essential. You can walk for about ten minutes before exercising. Or you can do some stretching. The idea is to get your blood pumping, start your heartbeat and breathing towards the rates you are going to ask of them. Stretching muscles after a warm-up will help prevent muscle tears and joint injury. When you finish all your exercises, cool off by taking a walk for about three minutes.

Shoulder Movements

Move your shoulder up and down as though you are shrugging. Keep your fists tightly closed. Inhale while lifting up the shoulders, and exhale as you lower them. Repeat this action ten times.

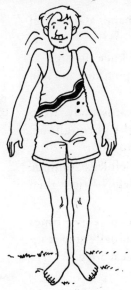

Toe Touching

(1) Stand erect, feet 12 inches apart, arms over head (2) Inhale, bend forward to touch floor between feet. Do not try to keep knees straight. (3) While exhaling, slowly return to the starting position. (4) Do this exercise five times to begin with, and gradually increase it to ten times by the weekend.

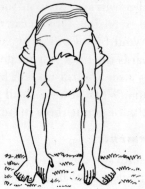

Knee Raising

(1) Stand erect, hands at sides, feet together.

(2) Raise right knee as high as possible, grasping knee and shin with hands.

(3) Pull leg towards body. Keep back straight throughout. Lower foot to floor.

(4) Repeat with left leg. Continue alternating legs — right then left.

(5) Do this two or three times initially. Gradually step it up to ten times each leg.

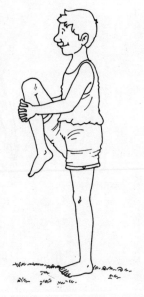

Side Bending

(1) Stand erect, feet 12 inches apart, hands at sides.

(2) Bend sideways from waist to left, keeping the back straight.

(3) Slide left hand down leg as far as possible.

(4) Return to the original position.

(5) Repeat this on the right side.

(6) Start off with five times each side, and increase it gradually to ten times.

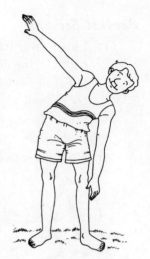

Arm Rotation

(1) Stand straight, feet 12 inches apart, arms at sides.

(2) With left arm, swing it in a circle, taking your arm in front, up, back, and down.

(3) Then reverse the direction.

(4) Repeat these circles with right arm.

(5) Do with both arms together in the same manner.

(6) Repeat this set of exercises ten times.

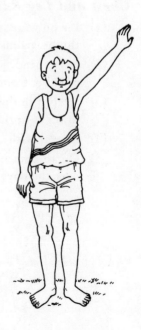

Partial Sit-ups

(1) Lie on your back with arms at the side of the body, palms facing downwards, feet stretched out together.

(2) Exhaling, slowly raise your shoulders and head, and try to look at your toes.

(3) Inhale as you lower your head and shoulders slowly to the floor.

(4) Do this exercise ten times.

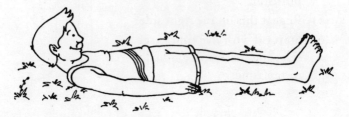

Chest and Leg Raising

(1) Lie on your stomach, arms by the sides, hands under thighs, palms pressing against thighs.

(2) Raise head, shoulders, and your left leg as high as possible from the floor.

(3) Keep it in that position for five seconds, then slowly lower it to the floor.

(4) Repeat with the other leg, the head and shoulders.

(5) Do this set of exercise initially thrice, increasing it over the days to ten.

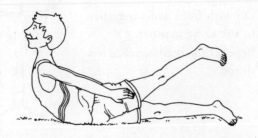

Lateral Leg Raising

(1) Lie on side, head resting on shoulder, legs straight, lower arm stretched out along floor to support the head, top arm on the side on the floor for balance.

(2) Slowly raise upper leg as high as possible, toes pointed.

(3) Slowly lower it to the starting position.

(4) Repeat on the other side.

(5) This set of exercises can be done five times to start with, gradually increasing it to 15 times.

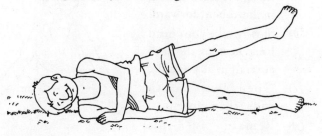

Spot Jogging

(1) Stand in one place of convenience, feet together, arms at sides.

(2) Run in place for about two minutes to start with.

(3) When running in place, lift knees forward, do not merely kick heels backwards.

(4) Keep the pace slow in the beginning and increase it gradually.

(5) Spot jogging should gradually be stretched to five minutes over time as a warm-up.

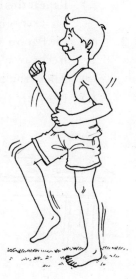

Special Areas Toning Up

The following exercises are easy-to-do exercises, meant to tone up and firm the body, while helping you to lose inches off your body. You can choose to do only certain exercises, if you are short of time, or do all of them, time permitting. Just don't push yourself though.

Neck

1. *(a)* Sit cross-legged on the floor, stomach drawn in, head bent forward.

   (b) Slowly take your head back, keeping the neck as straight as possible.

   (c) Open your mouth wide, then close it.

   (d) Remain in this position for ten seconds.

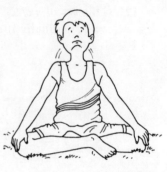

   (e) Repeat this exercise ten times. This will help to reduce the excess fat on the neck and jaws.

2. *(a)* Lie flat on a bench or settee with your head hanging freely away from the bench.

   (b) Allow the head to remain tilted downward.

   (c) Now lift your head slowly.

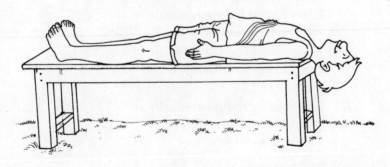

(*d*)   After about five seconds allow the head to drop back slowly to its original position.

(*e*)   Repeat this action ten times.

3.   (*a*)   Sit cross-legged on the floor, hands on your lap, head straight, tummy tucked in.

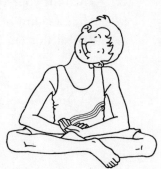

(*b*)   Rotate your head in a clockwise direction slowly five times.

(*c*)   Then rotate it anti-clockwise five times.

(*d*)   Try to stretch your neck as you do this rotation slowly.

Arms and Shoulders

1.   (*a*)   Stand erect with both arms raised over the head, palms pointing backwards.

(*b*)   Now turn the palms towards the front, and bring the hands down in front in line with the shoulders.

(*c*)   Now raise the arms over the head with palms in front.

(*d*)   Turn the palms upwards and bring down the arms at the sides in line with the shoulders.

(*e*)   Repeat this ten times.

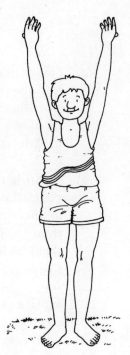

2. *(a)* Stand straight, with feet 12 inches apart.

   (b) Hold a pair of dumbbells in your hands and bend forward from your waist.

   (c) Then lift your arms sideways, your waist still bent.

   (d) After a count of ten, bring them down slowly.

   (e) Repeat this ten times.

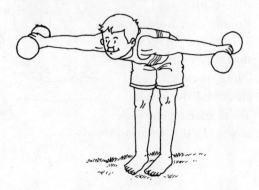

3. *(a)* Stand straight, with feet about 12 inches apart, fingers resting on shoulders, elbows out to sides at shoulder level.

   (b) Rotate both elbows in a circle, lowering them to sides then up front, then sideways to shoulder level.

   (c) Continue to circle thus, four circles as explained, and four circles in reverse direction.

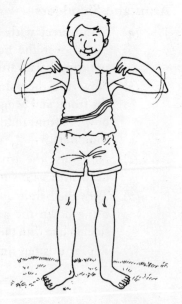

4. *(a)* Stand straight, right arm stretched out sideways at shoulder level, feet together.

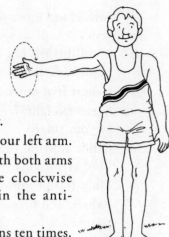

(b) Make circles with the arm, without bending your arm at the elbow.

(c) Repeat the same with your left arm.

(d) Repeat both actions with both arms together, first in the clockwise direction, and then in the anti-clockwise direction.

(e) Repeat this set of actions ten times.

Chest

1. *(a)* Stand straight with feet together, hands in front in line with the shoulders.

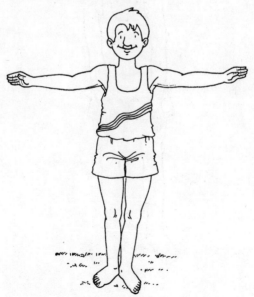

(b) Inhale, and move your hands to the sides at the same level.

(c) Hold this for few seconds, then exhale, and bring them back to the original position.

(d) Repeat five times.

2. (a) Stand straight, feet 12 inches apart, arms in front of your thighs.

(b) While inhaling, raise both your arms above your head at 45⁰ angle.

(c) Hold this position for a few seconds.

(d) Exhale, and bring back your arms to their original position.

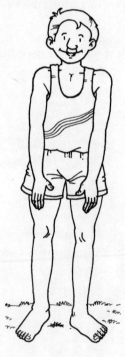

3.   *(a)*   Stand straight, feet 12 inches apart.

    (b)   Grasp the left wrist with the right palm, and the right wrist with the left palm.

    (c)   Raise them to shoulder level with the hands held in the same position.

    (d)   Push hard against each other, hold the wrists firmly.

    (e)   Repeat this 15 times.

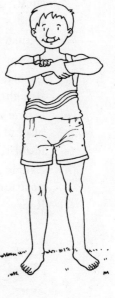

4.   *(a)*   Lie on your back, knees bent, feet on the floor.

    (b)   Keep the knees together, and holding dumbbells in your hands, stretch your arms sideways at shoulder level on the floor.

    (c)   Move your arms in the opposite directions over your

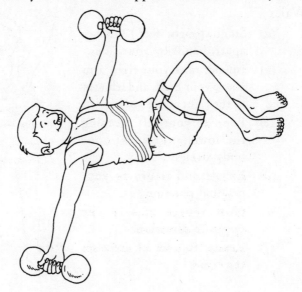

chest, scissors-like, ensuring that the arms do not bend at the elbow.

    (d) Return to the sides again, touching the floor.

    (e) Repeat this ten times.

5. *(a)* Lie flat on your back, hands on your thighs, feet straight and together.

    (b) Inhale and extend your hands upwards over your head at 45° angle.

    (c) Hold this position for a few seconds.

    (d) Exhale and then bring them back to their original position.

    (e) Repeat this ten times.

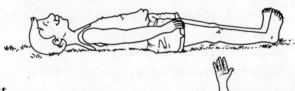

Waist

1. *(a)* Stand straight, feet 12 inches apart, hands by your sides.

    (b) Inhale, raise your right arm above your head, and left arm to the right across your waist.

    (c) Bend to your left, keeping the lower portion of your body straight.

    (d) Exhale and return to your original position.

    (e) Now repeat this in the opposite direction.

    (f) Repeat this set of exercises ten times.

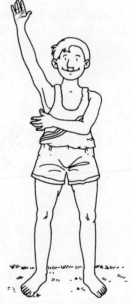

2. *(a)* Stand with feet 12 inches apart, hands by your sides.

   (b) Bend towards the right, as you inhale, and extend the left arm straight over your head, while you slide your right hand over your right leg.

   (c) Exhale and get back to the original position.

   (d) Repeat on the left side.

   (e) Do this exercise five times.

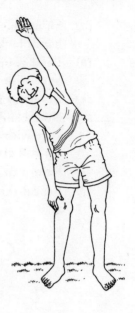

3. *(a)* Lie flat on your stomach, arms by your sides, feet together on the floor.

   (b) Gradually lift one foot from the ground as high as you can, keeping the knee straight.
   Bring the leg down. Repeat with other leg.

   (c) If you find the two steps easy to do, then raise your arms up as high as you can when you raise your legs.

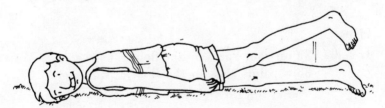

   (d) Hold this position for a few seconds and return to the original position. Rest for a few seconds.

   (e) Repeat this exercise five times.

4. *(a)* Sit on the floor, legs kept as wide apart as you can, hands locked together behind your head.

(b) Bend your body to the right trying to touch your knee with your elbow.

(c) Revert to the original position.

(d) Now bend to the left and try to touch your left knee with your left elbow, ensuring that the hands are still clasped behind your head.

(e) Return to your original position.

(f) Repeat this set of exercises ten times.

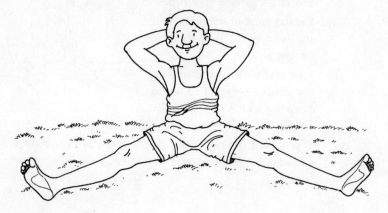

Hips

1. *(a)* Sit on your knees on the floor, both palms also on the floor, supporting your body.

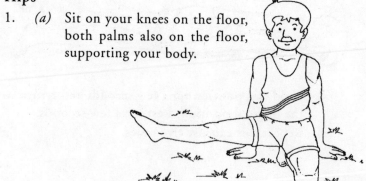

(b)   Extend your right leg to the side, foot resting on the floor.

(c)   Lift the leg as high as possible, then bring it back to the floor.

(d)   Repeat (c) ten times.

(e)   Repeat the whole presence with the left leg.

2.   (a)   Lit down flat on your back, hands stretched away from the body.

   (b)   Bend your knees and draw up your legs about six inches towards your buttocks.

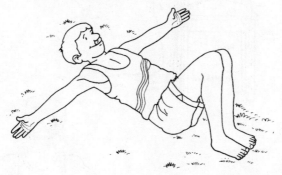

(c)   Lift your hips up, your feet and hands supporting your body weight.

(d)   Hold this position for a few seconds, then return to the original position.

3.   (a)   Stand straight, feet together, hands on the back of a chair for support.

   (b)   Gradually raise your right leg behind you, keeping the leg straight.

   (c)   Hold it to the count of ten, then return to the original position.

   (d)   Repeat with the left leg.

   (e)   Do this set of exercises ten times.

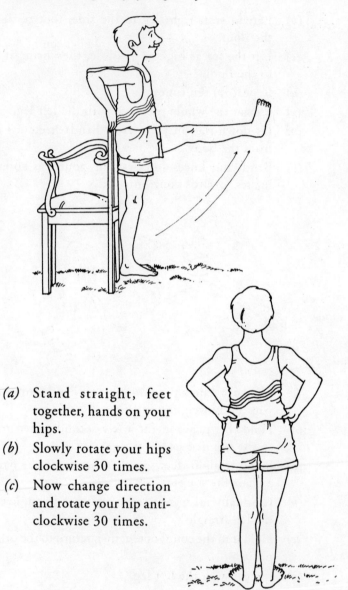

4. *(a)* Stand straight, feet together, hands on your hips.

    (b) Slowly rotate your hips clockwise 30 times.

    (c) Now change direction and rotate your hip anti-clockwise 30 times.

Abdomen

1. *(a)* Lie on your back, hands stretched out under the hips, legs together on the ground.

   (b) Lift both the legs slowly towards the ceiling, feet turned inwards, heels pointing outwards.

   (c) Then gradually lower them to 45⁰ angle, and hold them there to a count of ten.

   (d) Gradually bring down the legs to the floor.

   (e) Repeat this ten times.

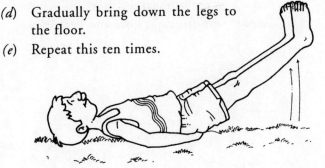

2. *(a)* Lie flat on your back, arms outstretched, palms on the ground.

   (b) Raise your left leg and bring it down to touch the fingers of your right hand.

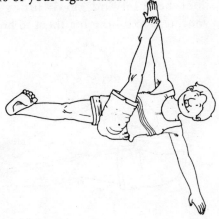

     (c)   Return to the original position.

     (d)   Repeat this with the right leg also.

     (e)   Repeat this set of exercises ten times.

3.   *(a)*   Lie flat on your back, arms clasped behind head, feet straight on the floor.

     (b)   Raise your neck, bend your left knee and try to touch the left knee with your right elbow.

     (c)   Return to the original position.

     (d)   Repeat with the right knee and left elbow.

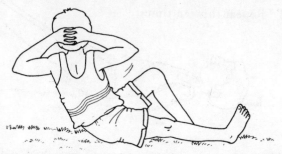

4.   *(a)*   Lie flat on your back, arms stretched out on the floor beyond your head, feet stretched out together.

     (b)   Now raise the upper part of your body from the floor, bend forward, slowly lifting your arms over your head and bringing them to hold the big toes.

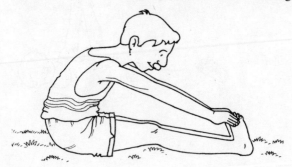

(c) Try to touch your knees with the chin.

(d) Return to the original position.

(e) Repeat this ten times.

Thighs

1. (a) Lie on the floor on your left side, right palm on the floor, resting the upper part of your body on the lower arm.

(b) Raise your right leg slightly off the floor and kick in the air.

(c) Repeat this ten times.

(d) Repeat with the other leg likewise.

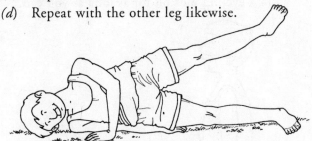

2. (a) Lie on your back, knees bent and feet on ground 12 inches apart, knees together, hands outstretched sideways on the floor.

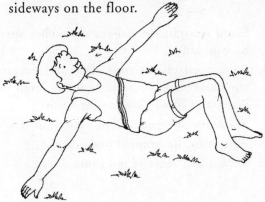

    (b)   Raise your buttocks off the floor, as high as possible, and hold it thus for a few seconds.

    (c)   Return to the original position.

    (d)   Repeat this exercise 15 times.

3.   *(a)*   Sit on the floor, palms resting on the floor near your body, legs stretched out in front.

    (b)   Move your palms a few inches behind you, and resting your weight on them and the buttocks, raise your feet six inches off the floor.

    (c)   Without the legs touching the floor, rotate the legs in a cycling motion for as long as you can.

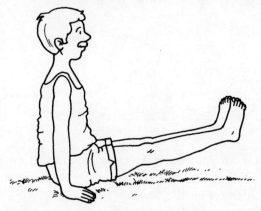

4.   *(a)*   Stand straight, feet about six inches apart, hands by your sides.

    (b)   Raise yourself on your toes, and keeping hands stretched out in front at shoulder level, bend your knees and slowly lower your body.

    (c)   Maintain this position to a count of ten.

    (d)   Return to the original position.

    (e)   Repeat this exercise ten times.

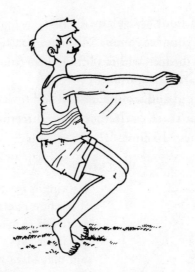

Feet and Ankles

1.   *(a)*   Sit on the floor, legs straight and about six inches apart, hands behind body for support, feet relaxed.

     (b)   Press toes away from body as far as possible.

     (c)   Bring toes towards body hooking feet as much as possible.

     (d)   Repeat this set of exercises 15 times.

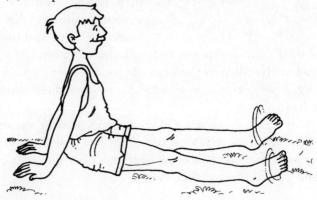

2.　*(a)*　Sit on floor as explained above.

　　(b)　Keep your feet about 14 inches apart.

　　(c)　Move the feet, without lifting them from the ground, in a circular motion.

　　(d)　Press out and around, and in and towards the body.

　　(c)　Repeat these circles in reverse direction also.

　　(f)　Do these 15 times.

WALKING

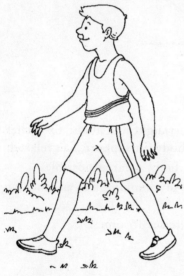

Walking is free, and it is one of the best overall workouts. A noted American heart specialist says, "It has been said that a five-mile walk will do more good to an unhappy but healthy adult than all the medicine and psychology in the world."

Now research emphasises the therapeutic value of walking, and shows how you can burn away a surprising number of unwanted calories in this way. Leave the car parked further away from your workplace, and walk that extra bit. Use stairs instead of lifts whenever you can, for you are giving your heart and legs a bonus of healthy exercise that you would not normally have had.

Walking provides many of the benefits of more strenuous activities, without much exertion. For this activity, you can progress at your own pace, no equipment is required, except a good pair of comfortable shoes.

Anyone should be able to find enough time to walk. Walk along the beach, walk around your building compound, or the mall, walk to the market, etc. Simply walk, be active, take up some active work. There is nothing difficult or faddish about walking, so it appeals to people of all ages. It keeps you slim, it helps beat stress—and its fun!

Walking has the advantage of being less prone to causing injuries as compared to other forms of exercise.

The benefits of walking are :

(a) It promotes more restful sleep.

(b) It helps in the reduction of tension and stress.

(c) It helps in reducing weight.

(d) Walking improves blood circulation, and is a good cardiovascular exercise.

(e) It improves the ability to take in oxygen.

(f) Researchers have found that walking for an hour a day decreases the risk of colon cancer by half, as it speeds digested foods through the body.

While walking, the following tips come in handy:

(a) Pull you chin in so that your ears are over your shoulders.

(b) Relax your shoulders.

(c) Concentrate on pulling your tummy in tight and pulled in.

(d) Walk with your arms swinging freely.

(e) Try landing strongly on your heels with your toes slightly lifted for a more powerful push off.

(f) Let your fingers relax.

(g) Hold your wrists straight.

(i) Breathe in deeply.

(j) Your stride should feel controlled and smooth.

(k) Keep your head up.

(l)   Be sure not to lean too far forward or back.

(m)   Wear shoes that are comfortable.

(n)   Observe carefully your surroundings, and enjoy the joys of nature.

(o)   Greet people you pass cheerfully, you will surprised at the number of appreciative smiles you get in return.

DANCING

Get your favourite tunes out and break a sweat! Tap dancing burns 400 calories in an hour while swing dancing burns 300 calories an hour.

Carry on dancing. It's fun, it's energetic, and it's friendly. All kinds of dancing provide good exercise, develop coordination of movement, flexibility, and can provide first class aerobic exercise.

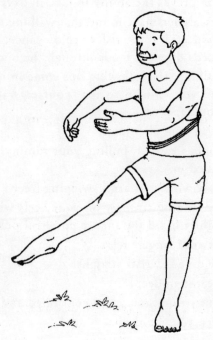

CYCLING

Cycling is a quick way of taking exercise that tones up the whole body, and burns off excess weight at the rate of 700 calories an hour! People are catching on to the idea that cycling is fun, healthy and altogether desirable for a host of reasons.

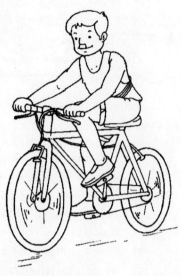

The heart, lungs and circulatory system have to work hard but without any strain being thrown upon joints as jogging does on the knee, ankle and hip joints of the not-so-young. The smooth rhythmic movement of pedalling is especially beneficial to people with painful joints which make even walking difficult. The cycle bears the weight, the muscles provide the power.

Why take up precious time going to a gym for aerobics when you can exercise your heart and legs with the exhilaration of sailing smoothly at a pace that makes you pant as little or much as you like?

Remember that cycling should be an enjoyable activity and not a painful chore.

SWIMMING

Swimming is a good way of exercising in the summer months. Beginners may face problems initially, but once a person learns to float on the water, he begins to enjoy himself.

Swimming is often recommended as an exercise to develop every muscle of the body in a harmonious way, and this includes your heart muscle.

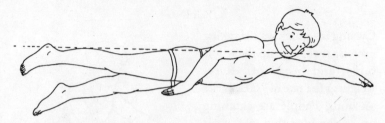

Swimming has a number of advantages over other forms of exercising:

(a) It is an excellent form of aerobics, and involves all the muscles which work at the same time, and then enhance the neuro-muscular coordination.

(b) Swimming gives a lot of relief from stress, and is being used in physiotherapy to revitalise injured muscles.

(c) It is a competitive as well as a recreational activity.

(d) Since the temperature of the water is lower than the body temperature, swimming strengthens the respiratory system, and the blood supply to the various parts improves.

(e) When painful joints in arthritic patients are supported in water, a degree of flexibility returns which is not normally seen in other situations.

(f) Swimming is strongly recommended for restoring muscle tone after childbirth.

(g) The gentle but rhythmic movement of leg muscles helps to avoid swollen veins and valves.